CW01507144

Cyborg Conception

Grace Halden

Cyborg Conception

Cultural and Critical Responses to Solo
Motherhood by Choice

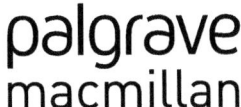

Grace Halden
School of Creative Arts, Culture and Communication
Birkbeck, University of London
London, UK

ISBN 978-3-031-59385-7   ISBN 978-3-031-59386-4   (eBook)
https://doi.org/10.1007/978-3-031-59386-4

This Palgrave Macmillan imprint is published by the registered company Springer Nature Switzerland AG.
The registered company address is: Gewerbestrasse 11, 6330 Cham, Switzerland

Paper in this product is recyclable.

For my children, Gabriel and Sebastian—with eternal love.

ACKNOWLEDGEMENTS

First and foremost, I am grateful to my parents, Joy and David Halden, who are both excellent examples of what it means to be selfless and devoted parents. I wouldn't have achieved anything at all if not for the love, support and guidance of my mum and dad. I also wish to thank my brother James Halden, who is an amazing uncle and has always been so supportive of my journey as a solo mother.

I am also so grateful to Lee Smith, my best friend. Not only has he read every single page of this book (three times), but he has been a reliable and generous friend for over fifteen years. Thank you to friends Janine Holness, Lauren Goodwin, Stephanie and Michael Scott, Kayleigh Kilbane, and Anne-Marie—all of whom appear somewhere in this book.

I am so fortunate to be part of such a warm, welcoming, and friendly solo mother community. I am particularly grateful to the women who volunteered to be interviewed for this book: Alexis, Eleni, Michelle, Nicola, Sam, Sarah A, Sarah B, Tamara, and Victoria; their generosity in sharing their experiences shows how incredibly supportive the Solo Mother by Choice (SMBC) community is. Over the last four years, I have also been lucky enough to find support and friendship in my solo mother friends Amy, Bonny, Emma, Karen, Lisa, Susan, Stephanie, and Stacey. Beyond the solo mother community, I have been helped by members of the donor conception community—notably Hayley King. I am grateful for the personal and professional assistance of the Donor Conception Network.

To all my colleagues at Birkbeck who have helped me with my writing, my ideas, grants, and applications, thank you. I am particularly indebted to Anthony Bale, Lisa Baraitser, Heike Bauer, Julia Bell, Suzannah Biernoff, Joseph Brooker, Luisa Calè, Richard Hamblyn, Esther Leslie, Roger Luckhurst, Sarah Marks, Silvia Posocco, Sue Wiseman, and Agnes Woolley. I wish to also thank two students: Jemma Walton, my PhD student whose work on reproduction is inspiring, and Siddharth Yadav, whose work on posthumanism really informed my own understanding. A special thank you to Anna Hartnell, who has been such an amazing mentor to me over the years and kindly offered feedback on early drafts of this book. Thank you also to Ana Parejo Vadillo, who is both a wonderful friend and a remarkable colleague.

Beyond Birkbeck, I wish to thank the excellent academic support around me, especially Harriet Barratt, Suzy Buckley, Peter Fifield, Zaina Mahmoud, Joanne Winning, and not forgetting Isabel Davis, who has continued to be such a figure of support in my life.

This book has emerged from my Cyborg Conception project, which was initially funded by the Birkbeck Wellcome Trust Institutional Strategic Support Fund (ISSF) (2020–2021). This fund has now closed, but when it was active it awarded millions to assist projects like mine. Without this financial support, I would not have been able to write this book.

I'm grateful to Palgrave for being so supportive and enthusiastic about *Cyborg Conception* and I'm so pleased that they welcomed the inclusion of personal accounts in this book because, as I argue in Chap. 5, the inclusion of lived experience is so important when writing about people, groups, and communities.

Of course, I thank my little sons—now five years old. My little fighters. I thank them for every glorious day I get to be a mother. I thank them for filling my home and life with joy and love.

That's a lot of people! I always knew the acknowledgement section would be packed. Writing a book is a bit like raising a baby—"it takes a village". I am grateful to every member of my village who has helped me both as a mother and as a writer.

I'll start this book in the same spirit as I finish it: being solo doesn't mean being alone.

CONTENTS

ABBREVIATIONS

DCN   Donor Conception Network
DCP   Donor Conceived Person
FDA   U.S. Food and Drug Administration
HFEA   Human Fertilisation and Embryology Authority
IUI   Intrauterine insemination
IVF   In-vitro fertilisation
MOT   Fertility "MOT": a test of reproductive health
NHS   National Health Service
NICU   Neo Natal Intensive Care
SMBC   Solo Mother by Choice
SMC   Single Mother by Choice
SPBC   Solo Parent by Choice

CHAPTER 1

Introduction

Abstract In *Cyborg Conception*, I consider the growing popularity of solo motherhood via gamete donation and how this type of "cyborg conception" is narrated in medicine, industry, fiction, and memoir. *Cyborg Conception* combines lived experience with scholarly research to present an overview of the solo motherhood phenomenon. In this introduction I explain the structure of the book and comment on the terminology and framework I will be employing throughout.

Keywords Assisted reproduction • Cyborg • Donna Haraway • Donor conception • Feminism • Gamete donation • Single mother • Solo mother • Structure • Terminology

REFLECTION

'It's ok to be a glow stick.' (A motivational quote I saw on the London Underground)

On the 15th of June 2017, I saw a poster on a tube train advertising babies. Of course, I am being facetious; what I actually saw as I sat on the London Underground on the way home from work was an invitation to a Fertility Fair on Harley Street. On it, a happy woman was holding a baby boy who pointed at me as if selecting me personally for motherhood. There was no man in the image; I, as a single woman, was being invited to try to conceive a child. At that moment, on the hot and crammed Circle Line train, I saw exactly what I had always wanted: I wanted to be a solo mother without a partner. It wasn't a backup plan, it wasn't a last resort, and the decision wasn't in any way sad, desperate, or painful.

I thought about the solo mother on the poster while I was travelling between Euston Square and Tower Hill; she made me remember that when I was a child I didn't fantasise about weddings or any form of cohabitation, but I did want to have a child. It was always just me and my baby—in play and in my dreams. I shaped my education and career around my quest to become a solo mother. The child pointing at me made me realise, in that precise moment, that I needed to enact my "Plan A" soon.[1] I was approaching 35. The child pointing at me wasn't inviting me to embark on a path I had only just considered. No, the child's podgy finger pointed accusingly at me amongst the throng of commuters and demanded to know why I dallied. 'You', he seemed to say, 'you're ready now.'

On the 25th of July 2018, almost a year after the Fertility Fair, I had intrauterine insemination with donor sperm—my second attempt. I didn't know it that day but my journey to being a mother of twin boys had started. It all sounds incredibly easy but it wasn't. Solo motherhood is not an easy pathway to traverse, and I have had to defend my lifestyle to others—both professionally as an academic working in the Medical Humanities and personally. I have found that I struggle to fit into pre-existing ideas of what it means to be a woman and a mother (especially as someone who doesn't align clearly with stereotypical ideas of gender, has not labelled myself with a sexuality, and is a mother to children who are fatherless in a social sense but have a genetic father through donation). I straddle so many ways of understanding gender, sex, and parenting but settle in no specific place nor category. It was my re-reading of Donna Haraway's 'Cyborg Manifesto' (1985) that made me realise that thinking in restrictive categories is not only unhelpful but that embracing the idea of the cyborg—a hybrid being of both literal and social reality—can 'suggest a way out of the maze of dualisms in which we have explained our bodies and our tools to ourselves' (1991, 181).

On the day I conceived my twins, I took a picture of the service information board at the entrance to Tower Hill station. Scrawled on it was a quote of the day. It read: 'It's ok to be a glow stick. Sometimes we need to break before we shine.' It is clichéd and trite but, nonetheless, I printed the picture and stuck it on the wall of my office. I think of it often and keep it in my head as a mantra. It's ok to be a glow stick, it's ok to be a cyborg, it's ok to break boundaries and binaries and convention. It is through doing this that new ways of thinking and being can shine.

Introduction: Cultural and Critical Responses to Solo Motherhood by Choice

Reproduction is one of the most fundamental biological functions of living organisms; for humans, sexual reproduction is not only a pathway to genetic offspring, but—for many—a rite of passage. The importance of reproductive health is underscored in society yet family planning discourse is commonly limited to heteronormative nuclear family constructs. Donor gamete conception (donation of sperm and eggs) has enabled the development of diverse family models for years. Today, many women are choosing to conceive solo through donor conception, a decision which is lauded as empowering but also demonised as unethical. *Cyborg Conception* considers how the rise of solo mothers by choice (often abbreviated as SMBC) through donor conception (sperm, donor eggs, and/or donor embryos) is the realisation of a radical cyborg feminism made popular by Donna Haraway in her 'Cyborg Manifesto' (1985). In short, Haraway imagines the cyborg as the disruption of traditional ways of understanding natural/ unnatural, organic/technological, and other related dichotomies. Haraway's Manifesto was published in the same decade that the organisation 'Single Mothers by Choice' (1981) was formed. *Cyborg Conception* identifies solo mothers as women who exist in a space beyond binarity (male/female, dual-rearing dynamic) and heteronormative discourse; the solo mother represents, among other diverse family constructions (such as same-sex couples and throuples), a critical intervention in the dominant narrative of the nuclear family which defines the "ideal" reproductive model. In this book, I consider the growing popularity of solo motherhood via gamete donation and how this type of "cyborg conception" is narrated in contemporary culture.

The full title of Haraway's manifesto is 'A Cyborg Manifesto: Science, Technology, and Socialist-Feminism in the Late Twentieth Century', and was originally published in *Socialist Review* in 1985 and then republished in her book *Simians, Cyborgs and Women: The Reinvention of Nature* in 1991. Haraway's essay is considered a 'legend of late 20th-century scholarship' (Hayles 1999, 159). Although it was first written in the 1980s (and despite Haraway's work no longer engaging with the cyborg and her criticisms about reproduction itself), the Manifesto retains cultural currency and is integral to modern understandings of the cyborg. As literary critic N. Katherine Hayles remarks:

> 'A Manifesto for Cyborgs' remains vitally important, perhaps even more so than in 1985, the original publication date. The issues have morphed in significant ways, but the ethical drive and social commitment that galvanized readers then were never more necessary. With the hindsight of twenty years later, the wonder is not that the article appears dated but rather that it remains remarkably prescient in many of its concerns. (2006, 159)

I will return in more detail to Haraway in Chap. 2 when I explore the history and definitional development of the cyborg. In this introductory chapter, I want to look more broadly at the surrounding field—one Hayles and Haraway are perhaps most famously known for—that of posthumanism. The cyborg is a central figure within posthumanism because both concepts broadly contend with the reimagining of traditional boundaries between the natural and the artificial. Of course, I am not looking at the stereotypical idea of cyborg in science fiction, so we are going to leave imaginings of Robocop at the door. Instead, I am engaging with a theoretical model which argues that human reproduction is increasingly framed by technology and through this—potentially "posthuman" evolution— ideas of what reproduction means have been diversified, which has also helped to diversify how family is understood conceptually.

Posthumanism, as a philosophy, responds to the drive to rethink what human is and what human means at a time of intense scientific, medical, and technological developments which are viewed as radically impacting the human experience and human world. For the purposes of this book, one example of technological impact is assisted reproduction and how developments in this field of biotechnology are reframing how conception occurs. Broadly, the term posthuman is utilised to cover many different concepts and has been defined and characterised differently by various scholars. Robert Pepperell aptly notes that the term posthuman can 'describe a number of things at once' and, in part, can refer to the 'general convergence of biology and technology to the point where they are increasingly becoming indistinguishable' (1995, iv). For the timeline of this book, which identifies a turning point in assisted reproduction in 1978 and the growing popularisation of donor conception in mainstream culture from the 1980s onwards (as noted in detail in Chap. 2), it is notable that the roots of posthumanism in academic discourse are said to originate in the 1970s (see Ferrando 2013, 26–7).[2] Rather than positioning the human as something historic and the posthuman as a futuristic development, Hayles complicates the timeframe of the posthuman as evident in the title of her book *How We Became Posthuman* (1999). For Hayles there are no 'sharp breaks' with posthuman emergence; instead the posthuman has simply 'reinscribed traditional ideas and assumptions' (1999, 6).

I play with similar ironies in my title *Cyborg Conception* because, as I shall evidence, I do not imagine cyborg conception as a future state but a current and ever evolving one. I am not the first person to use the term cyborg conception. In Robbie Davis-Floyd's and Joseph Dumit's edited collection *Cyborg Babies: From Techno-Sex to Techno-Tots* (1998), they dedicate a whole section of their book to cyborg conception, focusing on early technological mediation in reproduction such as in-vitro fertilisation (IVF) which was first achieved in 1978 with the birth of Louise Brown. I am doing something different. I focus not so much on the cyborg as a 'technological artefact' but as a 'cultural icon', to borrow Hayles' phrasing (1999, 2), and in terms of its metaphorical significance (in Haraway's understanding). This means I am far more interested in how the cyborg and SMBC are viewed and understood culturally rather than in how the science works.

I also don't imagine cyborg conception as a moment of cultural shock. My approach imagines the cyborg as pervasive. Therefore, I avoid reading assisted reproduction and associated technologies (from freezing gametes to IVF) as mere aids. Instead of focusing on the idea of prosthesis (traditionally viewed as an external and artificial part, tool or device to replace ordinary human function, such as an artificial limb), I understand reproductive assistance and mediation as ubiquitous: as part of human evolution. I agree with Cary Wolfe who notes that the posthuman, in part, helps us appreciate that the human 'has coevolved with various forms of technicity and materiality' (2009, xxv). Francesca Ferrando is also right when she remarks that 'Technology is a trait of the human outfit' (2013, 28). Such articulations chime with Hayles' understanding that the posthuman is human and technology 'seamlessly articulated' (1999, 3). This is why I avoid thinking of cyborg as the utilisation of external tools and instead view the human and technology working together in symbiosis. I understand that this viewpoint is somewhat against the grain. Technology is often imagined as an external force that disrupts or invades the natural human state (which is often presented as sacred) and mutates the natural into something else (usually something negative). This "something else" is often framed as unnatural or artificial, and decidedly a problematic modern phenomenon. Instead, I suggest that if we think of both the body and technology as matter then we start at a more neutral place in which hybridity is less jarring and more collaborative.[3] Thinking of the body and technology as matter working cohesively is helpful when thinking about the cyborg. Thinking also that this collaboration is an historical phenomenon (we have always used tools) resists the urge to think that technological assistance/mediation is something new.

I believe that for a long time reproduction has been mediated and assisted in various ways. Hayles notes that the posthuman marks how 'the human is giving way to a different construction', and I argue that traditional reproduction is increasingly 'giving way' to cyborg conception. The "manipulation" of reproduction is commonplace and across a wide spectrum from fertility diets (e.g. increasing Omega-3 fatty acids to improve egg quality), to "over the counter" supplements, to prescribed Gonal-F injections for follicle stimulation. When Hayles writes that 'cyborgs actually exist' she refers to 'technical' cyborgs that have that literal melding of artificial parts and organic components (such as the pacemaker) and 'metaphorical cyborgs' like the 'computer keyboarder' (1999, 115). This is similar to how cyborg conception is viewed as a purely technical act in *Cyborg Babies*. However, I add a third layer here when discussing cyborg conception: how making, gestating, birthing, rearing, and reproducing is being rethought conceptually. This marks a more "naturalised" hybridity that is not necessarily observable as cyborg for it lacks the obvious technological connections (lack of visual melding such as artificial limbs and lack of observable engagement with technology such as computer usage).

In this book I present SMBC as an explicit example of cyborg conception through a tripartite understanding of the cyborg as technologically mediated, metaphorical, and social (which I will explain in the next chapter). But, in brief, gametes (which are biological components), become used like technology to enable "solo conception". In a purely functional sense, IVF and IUI (intrauterine insemination) take reproductive cells outside the body and use technology to assist these cells in their original solitary function—which is to fertilise.[4] In this respect, the gamete can be viewed as a cog within a technological process without undermining the significance of what DNA and conception means to human beings themselves. This new augmented way of conceiving contributes to new understandings of family construction and we find new (sometimes ironic) language emerging, such as "conceiving solo". The solo women who conceive alone via gamete donation demonstrate literal technological mediation, metaphorical one-parent reproduction, and the social reality of a "fatherless" family. SMBC is not the only way conception is cyborg, but solo conception is a powerful example of this manifestation. Further, as I shall illustrate throughout this book, SMBC is often demonised as a pathway because it is often viewed as challenging the "natural", traditional, and "ideal" heterosexual nuclear family model.

I am not proposing that the solo mother by choice—whom we must remember is primarily a woman who needs assistance to make her family—is directly engaged in a posthuman movement or would define herself as posthuman or cyborg. Instead, I suggest terms like posthuman and cyborg—sometimes considered to be scary—are not looming future catastrophes but shifts that have happened and are continuing to happen. Often, we do not notice this 'becoming posthuman' (to borrow Hayles' term) because we perhaps imagine the cyborg to be something visually sensational, socially disruptive, or linked to apocalyptic imagination. Instead, I argue that not only is cyborg conception happening but also that it is helping us to rethink once restrictive ideas of family, parenting, and kinship in very important and positive ways.

In Chap. 2, I will unpick the development of the cyborg as a term and as a concept and lean on the work of Haraway who speaks of the cyborg as a boundary breaking feminist icon.[5] I will also consider the importance of the 1980s to both the SMBC movement and our cultural appreciation of the cyborg. However, before we get there, I want to introduce another feminist writer who reflects on the cyborg—Mary Harrington. In 2023, writer Mary Harrington published *Feminism Against Progress* in which she argues that the pursuit of feminist liberation has been confounded by the simultaneous development of 'progressive' technologies (such as the contraceptive pill) which have led to a detachment of women from nature and their own bodies as they become increasingly commodified as cyborg. Where Haraway sees liberation in the cyborg as binary busting and boundary blurring, Harrington sees a dystopian future (2023, 17). Posthumanism is, for Harrington, the eradication of difference and the undermining of what it means to be human; whereas, I view it as a celebration of the human, an homage to the human, and a collaboration of human and environment.

For Mary Harrington, "cyborg feminism" sees the establishment of 'personhood on the same terms as men' but problematically achieved because it is 'underwritten by technology' which, in turn, risks creating an 'atomized, sexless, liberal person' (Harrington and Allen 2022). Harrington dates the cyborg era to the 1970s and the legalisation of abortion in America, controversially arguing that technological aids such as the contraceptive pill are problematic transhumanist developments that render the body 'a problem to be solved' (Harrington and Allen 2022). In my view, this approach misses the many other benefits of the contraceptive pill—a pharmaceutical used by non-heterosexual women for a range of issues (I use it despite not being at risk from unwanted pregnancy). For Harrington, the cyborg is a problem and has positioned women's personhood as 'predicated on and inseparable from certain technologies' (Harrington and Allen 2022). *Feminism Against Progress* critiques the argument that the cyborg promises 'freedom' and 'progress' by arguing that the cyborg has replaced the ambitions of feminism but without promoting the interests of women (Harrington 2024). Therefore, it is argued that the cyborg marks the end of "true" feminism. I not only question what the "interests of women are" but what women are included under this banner because those who are not in heterosexual relationships benefit from assisted reproductive technologies, without which they could not create a family. For SMBC the cyborg is not only in the "interests of women" but helps realise the freedom and progress ushered in by the previous feminist waves. Harrington and I are united on the fact that the cyborg impacts reproduction today, but we part ways on how we view this impact. For me, SMBC represent how new conception options mean women have greater autonomy over their bodies and reproductive options. While *Cyborg Conception* does not engage deeply in feminist theory and its movements, it frames cyborg conception as demonstrating reproductive freedom across gender, sex, race, class, and sexuality.[6] This book should be seen as part of the unfinished project of feminism; it is itself a feminist book, focusing on the prioritisation of opportunities and fair treatment of women outside of the male/female framed ideal reproductive arrangement.

Cyborg Conception traces four major influences on how SMBC is narrativised in the contemporary: the field of moral philosophy, the reproductive medicine industry, popular culture, and stories of lived experience. Chapter 2 builds on the cyborg introduced in this chapter by exploring different definitions and understandings of the cyborg. I establish how I am using the term cyborg conception in light of three major movements in the 1980s: Haraway's 'social reality' of the cyborg, interest in goddess feminism, and increased interest in SMBC. Following the historical framing of the SMBC as cyborg, in Chap. 3 I pivot from theory to examine real-world implications of the SMBC by focusing on how she is represented in anti-donation discourse and in fertility clinics. My intent here is to explore how in moral philosophy and in clinical practice SMBC are viewed as occupying a liminal space in which they do not represent the parenting "norm". SMBC often do not fit the profile of women seeking fertility treatment (often partnered infertile women) and therefore are often underrepresented (and certainly underfunded) as patients. Moreover, I consider how anti-donation debate can present solo motherhood via donation as an inadequate parenting model. Despite the liberation associated with the cyborg mother in Chap.2, in Chap. 3 I show the SMBC as struggling for positive representation due to the dominance of the nuclear family dynamic as the ideal parenting formation. If the "normal" family and "happily ever after" are traditionally depicted as heterosexual and coupled (a princess waiting for her prince), then how are SMBC presented in mainstream film, television, and literature? In Chap. 4, I look at some popular examples in fiction storytelling in which the SMBC is depicted as either a demonised single mother or as a redeemed co-parent within a new romance. I find that the fictionalised SMBC is largely reduced to stereotype and identify a trend in which the solo mother becomes a successful parent once refolded into the male/female nuclear parent binary. Moving away from fiction, in Chap. 5 I turn to consider real-life accounts from women who have chosen to become solo mothers via gamete donation. I delve deeply into the importance of personal storytelling when looking at the narratives of lived experience by those directly within the donor conception community. Finally, in the conclusion I reflect on the terminology associated with SMBC and how the ongoing stigmatisation of the single mother and the woolly issue of "choice" has complicated what it means for women outside of the "choice community" to have reproductive autonomy.

Combined, these topics offer an interdisciplinary exploration of literature, science, technology, philosophy, law, art, and media in relation to solo motherhood. There is an inevitable bleeding between each chapter as ideas and conceptions weave from clinical spaces to popular cultural understandings. By moving from the specialist spaces of the fertility clinic to the broader public-engaged spaces of fiction and personal storytelling, we see certain issues sustained—such as prioritisation of the heterosexual nuclear family. As a SMBC myself, it would be disingenuous not to identify my own experiences so each chapter will begin with a personal reflection before moving on to an academic analysis of each theme.

A Note About Terminology

In this book, I will be using specific terminology. As I have already noted, SMBC stands for Solo Mother/s by Choice (and Solo Motherhood by Choice). For some individuals Solo Parenthood by Choice (SPBC) is preferred. As SMBC is a commonly accepted term in both the donor conception community and the assisted reproduction industry, this is the term and abbreviation I will use for the most part. In terms of defining SMBC, they are often defined as 'neither cohabiting nor married and the conception is intended' (Hayford and Guzzo 2015, 71). Solo mother Mikki Morrissette offers a more nuanced definition: 'women who consciously and responsibly choose single motherhood after asking serious questions about what that lifestyle means, for self and child [...] someone who proactively seeks to become a nurturing mother on her own' (2008, xiii). For clarity, in this book, the term SMBC will refer specifically to solo motherhood via gamete donation in which the mother conceives, gestates, and births as a solo parent using donor gametes (sperm or the double donation of sperm and egg or embryo donation). Solo motherhood via adoption, surrogacy, and solo fatherhood have their own triumphs, challenges, and complexities in terms of journey and narrativisation; it would be a disservice to these unique forms of family construction for me to cover all forms of solo parenting. As I am a solo mother through gamete donation, I am focusing on this particular pathway.

I prefer the terms "assisted reproduction" and "alternative insemination" to "artificial insemination" for, as Naomi Cahn notes in *Test Tube Families*, 'alternative insemination' is 'more value-neutral' (2009, 10). Assisted reproduction as a term incorporates intrauterine insemination, in vitro fertilisation, intracervical insemination, and intracytoplasmic sperm injection (abbreviated as IUI, IVF, ICI, ICSI, respectively). While sperm donation is the most common way for solo women to conceive, this book does not forget other pathways such as double donation and embryo donation even though it might not mention these routes directly. My focus in this book is on critical and cultural narratives about solo motherhood so, although this book discusses assisted reproduction, I will not discuss the specific reproductive pathways in detail. Further, I am aware that some people born as biological women may identify as transgender, non-binary, and/or would prefer the neutral term "parent" over "mother". Indeed, many solo mothers/parents by choice are within the LGBTQ+ community. When I refer to women throughout this book, I do so due to the necessitation of talking about biologically female reproductive processes.

Primarily, I will be talking about formal gamete donation via regulated banks and clinics in the United Kingdom because laws on donor conception vary from country to country. Although I acknowledge and discuss informal pathways (such as sourcing a known donor through sites like Facebook)[7] and other industry systems in countries like Australia, America, and Japan, it will mainly be the UK's formal donor conception system discussed here. Regulatory practices differ wildly; in the UK, a formal sperm donor can assist up to ten families and must be a known or identity release donor (this means the donor-conceived child can learn the donor's identity when the child reaches the age of eighteen). I am sensitive to the trauma donor-conceived people have experienced historically regarding lack of transparency over their origins and lack of access to donor medical data. Before 2005, in the UK, it was common for donations to be completely anonymous and for children to be raised without knowledge of their donor conception; since the regulatory changes in 2005, openness and honesty are recommended by leading industry informants including the Donor Conception Network and the Human Fertilisation and Embryology Authority. While it is my belief that the global industry should attempt to reach a universal standard of care in which completely anonymous donations are phased out and a global limit of assisted families per donor is established, this book focuses on SMBC in critical thinking and cultural works and therefore does not deal specifically with issues of regulation nor experiences of donor-conceived people—which would need a bespoke book with contributions from those with lived experience. I encourage readers to seek out the testimonies of donor-conceived people to better understand the importance of regulated, non-anonymous donations as well as the importance of raising children with awareness of their donor conception.[8] In the following footnote I supply a range of references that should be used as a starting point to become familiar with the experiences of donor-conceived people.[9] My intent in writing this book is to specifically identify dominant narratives shaped in the media, academia, and popular culture surrounding the family pathway of solo motherhood.

Finally, a note about the use of the term "solo mother" over "single mother". Reproduction has always been understood in binary terms as male/female and egg/sperm. With the innovation of assisted reproductive technologies and treatment for same-sex couples, an additional binary of heterosexual/homosexual is often added to articulate the different pathways of reproduction for these family formations. SMBC are also defined in a binary: while everyone else in the clinic is *paired* in their reproduction journey, SMBC are the opposite, they are *solo*. However, for many critics, the designation commonly used for these women—solo mothers/parents by choice—is problematic. The distinction between single and solo and the addition of 'by choice' is often misconstrued as a classist act to separate solo parents through gamete donation from the stigmatised single mother who has been demonised in society and culture for centuries. I disagree with Jane D. Bock when she notes in her article on legitimacy and single mothers that

> [b]y appropriating the term single mother by choice (SMC),[10] midlife middle-class single women implicitly claim their entitlement to make this decision. The SMC label serves as a tool to indicate their place at the top of the single-parent hierarchy and implies that other single mothers do not enter parenthood by choice or, at least, not by a choice as responsible as their own (see Trent and Crowder 1997). Thus, the label itself serves to separate this population from other single mothers, those who allegedly are the "real" problem. (2000, 64)

Narratives which pit single mothers and solo mothers against each other with stereotypes connecting single mothers to poverty and solo mothers to privilege are problematic (another unhelpful binary). Bock notes 'middle-class status and fiscal capability legitimise the mothers and the decision to mother; unlike welfare-dependent mothers, SMCs can fully take on the instrumental responsibilities of child care' (2000, 73). Bock's article was published in 2000 and today many SMBC seek donation pathways through at-home insemination and combine government support with low-wage or part-time earnings. If there was a divide between the "poor" single mother and the "financially privileged" solo mother by choice, this divide is no longer so deeply contrasted.

The idea of "choice" as linked specifically to a certain type of one-parent family (e.g. via gamete donation) comes with inherent challenges.

Not only does the inclusion of choice in SMBC (unintentionally) suggest that, in contrast, single women are circumstantially saddled with children, but that there are real questions about when, how, and to whom these "choices" apply. While more women are turning to DIY insemination and the image of the SMBC as being financially privileged is changing, the fact remains that treatment within a clinic is expensive and is simply a choice that many cannot make. Furthermore, those who choose this path are often already enveloped in supportive structures and do not necessarily have to contend with religious or cultural restraints. It is important not to lose sight that the inclusion of the word "choice" does not mean that this is an easy choice nor one available to every woman equally.

I suggest that the problem with the designation SMBC is not only with how the word "choice" is used but also with how women are defined by relationship status. Solo is a neutral term which could mean the mother is dating or single but is—for whatever reason—without a co-parent. In the conclusion, I outline in detail why solo, not single, should be used for all mothers who parent alone, regardless of their conception history and relationship status. I also suggest that the word "choice" should be reconsidered and suggest that "solo parenthood through donation" (SPD) may be a preferable term. That said, over the next few chapters, I will differentiate between single mothers and solo mothers to intentionally highlight the demonisation of single/solo mothers across what I call a "spectrum of selfishness" in which on one end there are women who are presented as accidentally parenting solo (by circumstance) and on the other end women who are presented as recklessly parenting alone (by choice). No matter where a woman is on that spectrum, they face the same ethical criticism: the argument that it is better to raise a child in a heterosexual, nuclear family co-parenting dynamic than any other.[11] It is, therefore, important not to think about the ways in which these women are different (privileged/underprivileged) but to focus on the ways in which patriarchal structures, misogynistic mindsets, and heteronormative ideals work collectively to argue that romantically single women have an obligation not to parent solo. In such debates, in which certain women are obligated not to conceive, there is no "privilege" dividing us; the discrimination train does not have "privileged" and "underprivileged" compartments. We are all the same class.

Notes

1. Throughout, I refer to Plan A and Plan B as routes commonly discussed in the SMBC community. Plan A tends to refer to those who wanted to conceive with a sperm donor from the outset, while Plan B refers to those who wanted a different family setup originally (e.g. a coparenting romantic relationship) but needed to choose donor conception when that ideal did not pan out.

2. Francesca Ferrando identifies Ihab Habib Hassan in "Prometheus as Performer: Toward a Posthumanist Culture?" 1977, as responsible for the coinage of posthumanism.

3. Reflection on matter in contrast to the use of the natural is inspired by Olga Goriunova's presentation on mapping data processes at Terramorphosis II: Patterns Symposium—26 January at Birkbeck College, University of London.

4. This does not mean that we should imagine gametes as mere "things" without consideration of their enormous impact on how the resulting individual will consider their construction and identity. However, at the most basic level, a gamete is a reproductive cell within an organism in which its only function is fertilisation. Moreover, gametes are data (chromosomal data, genetic data) and provide information language; as Biologist Leroy Hood summarised, 'biology is an information science.' For Hood, the genome is a 'rosetta stone' (Hood 1998).

5. Haraway's Manifesto is not just feminist but a call for action and a demand for the rejuvenation of the movement itself. Because Haraway's work was a starting point for my thinking on the cyborg, and because much has been written on Haraway's reading of socialist-feminism, it may seem obvious for this book to argue that solo mothers through gamete (sperm and/or egg) donation (formally known as Solo Mothers by Choice, SMBC) who conceive, birth and raise children alone represent feminist achievement. This is not what I am arguing. In fact, as Su Holmes notes in the article 'The Solo Mum, Feminism and the Negotiation of "Choice"', many SMBC do not recognise 'the decision to become a solo mum as one that emerged out of female empowerment or agency' (2018). As a phenomenon, the rise of SMBC does something more complex than highlight a feminist realisation of social equality of the sexes through the establishment of personal, economic, and political parity. SMBC marks a divergence from restrictive ways of thinking about family construction at a time in which there are cultural shifts which unpick rigid binaries relating to how sex, gender, and sexuality are experienced.

6. Much has been written about solo/single motherhood and feminism (Morrissette (2008), Mattes (1997), Sloane (2007)). Much has also been

written on the cyborg and feminism—Donna Haraway and Mary Harrington are just two voices in this conversation. There is space in this field for a specific book that explores the complications of feminism (and its numerous forms) and the complexity of the solo and single mother divide in society, culture, and clinical spaces. Tracing the development of SMBC from the 1980s to the present covers different feminist waves and feminist perspectives such as the second and third feminist waves and emergent movements such as radical feminism, liberal feminism, socialist feminism, and postfeminism. In terms of motivation and context they differ in approach and ambition but—broadly speaking—all advocate for reproductive and bodily autonomy, support reproductive justice and equality (reproductive equality across gender, race and class), and resist the narrative of motherhood as an idealised "success" story for women and critique any form of coercive reproduction. This book is not intended to critique solo motherhood through a feminist lens. However, I do acknowledge that SMBC is possible due to the advances made by feminism (e.g. opportunities for women to work, access childcare, access benefits—such as child benefits—and access the National Health Service in the UK, etc.). I also acknowledge that the SMBC continues to be stigmatised by the belief that successful mothering exists in heterosexual two-parent constructions which shows that more work needs to be done. Although this book is not a feminist reading of SMBC, I hope that at its heart it contributes to one of the core themes of feminist discourse: that reproductive autonomy remains one of the most important issues facing women.

7. While informal donation carries the benefit of raising a child with a known donor, there are potential legal issues with this route as the donor can request parental rights at any time. This route is complex and should be explored independently in a dedicated volume. In this book, I am focusing on formal donations as I am exploring, in part, the clinical space and treatment options.

8. Some SMBC will have used anonymous donors, unregulated donors, or those with large global limits. These decisions may have been made before the regulation changes in 2005, or they may have been necessitated by the laws of the country in which they sought treatment. My comments here are not intended as judgement on individual choices but instead to highlight what, ideally, should happen in the global donor conception market. Ideally, gamete banks and clinics should offer known or identity release donors and all donations should have a fixed global limit.

9. To hear a range of personal stories by donor-conceived people visit the following websites: *We Are Donor Conceived* (2023), *The Donor Conceived Community* (2023), and *The Donor Conception Network* (2023) (specifi-

cally the page on personal stories). The following documentaries highlight the importance of non-anonymous donations and also donation limits: Barry Stevens' *Offspring* (2001); Jerry Rothwell's *Donor Unknown* (2010); Lucy Paplinska's *Sperm Donors Anonymous* (2015). See also the podcast *You Look Like Me* by Louise McLoughlin (2020). For research on the importance of non-anonymous donations and for better understanding of the interest donor-conceived people have in identifying and locating donor relatives, see the following research: Ravitsky (2012), Hertz et al. (2013) and Adams and Allan (2013). I am unable to link every resource available but offer these materials as a starting point. I have tried to offer sources beyond the UK to ensure diversity of experiences. Information on these sources can be found in the Reference List.

10. SMC and SMBC are often used interchangeably. SMC was coined by Mattes to refer to Single Mother by Choice; SMBC refers to Solo Mother by Choice. Mattes intended SMC to encompass different types of single mothers whereas SMBC tends to refer to solo mothers via gamete donation.

11. The exception seems to be the widow who is often presented as a victim and therefore a justified single mother through no choice and tragic circumstances. I am indebted to Dr Anna Hartnell for this observation.

References

Adams, D., and S. Allan. 2013. Building a Family Tree: Donor-Conceived People, DNA Tracing and Donor 'Anonymity'. *Australian Journal of Adoption* 7 (2): 1–16.

Bock, J.D. 2000. Doing the Right Thing? Single Mothers by Choice and the Struggle for Legitimacy. *Gender and Society* 14(1): 62–86. http://www.jstor.org/stable/190422. Accessed March 4, 2021.

Cahn, N.R. 2009. *Test Tube Families. Why the Fertility Market Needs Legal Regulation.* New York: New York University Press.

Davis-Floyd, R., and J. Dumit, eds. 1998. *Cyborg Babies: From Techno-Sex to Techno-Tots.* London: Routledge.

Ferrando, F. 2013. Posthumanism, Transhumanism, Antihumanism, Metahumanism, and New Materialisms Differences and Relations. *Existenz* 8 (2): 26–32.

Haraway, D. 1991. A Cyborg Manifesto: Science, Technology, and Socialist-Feminism in the Late Twentieth Century. In *Simians, Cyborgs, and Women: The Reinvention of the Nature*, 149–182. New York: Routledge.

Harrington, M. 2023. *Feminism Against Progress.* Croydon: Forum.

———. 2024. We Already Live in the Cyborg Era. *Reactionary Feminist.* https://reactionaryfeminist.substack.com/about. Accessed January 30, 2024.

Harrington, M., and Allen, E. 2022. Cyborg Feminism. *Public Discourse*, December 8. https://www.thepublicdiscourse.com/2022/12/86306/. Accessed January 30, 2024.

Hayford, S.R., and K.B. Guzzo. 2015. The Single Mother by Choice Myth. *Contexts: Understanding People in Their Social Worlds* 14: 70–72.

Hayles, N.K. 1999. *How We Became Posthuman: Virtual Bodies in Cybernetics, Literature, and Informatics*. Chicago: University of Chicago Press.

———. 2006. Unfinished Work: From Cyborg to Cognisphere. *Theory, Culture & Society* 23 (7–8): 159–166. https://doi.org/10.1177/026327640606922. Accessed November 22, 2023.

Hertz, R., M.K. Nelson, and W. Kramer. 2013. Donor Conceived Offspring Conceive of the Donor: The Relevance of Age, Awareness, and Family Form. *Social Science and Medicine* 86: 52–65. https://doi.org/10.1016/j.socscimed.2013.03.001. Accessed January 12, 2021.

Holmes, S. 2018. The Solo Mum, Feminism and the Negotiation of 'Choice.' *Elsevier*. https://doi.org/10.1016/j.wsif.2018.04.007. Accessed November 12, 2023.

Hood, L.H. 1998. Keynote Address: Impact of Biotechnology and Environmental Research on Science and Society in the 21st Century. US Department of Energy. National Research Council (US). Serving Science and Society in the New Millenium: DOE's Biological and Environmental Research Program. Washington (DC): National Academies Press (US). https://www.ncbi.nlm.nih.gov/books/NBK230603/. Accessed March 12, 2024.

Mattes, J. 1997. *Single Mothers by Choice: A Guidebook for Single Women Who Are Considering or Have Chosen Motherhood*. New York: Three Rivers Press.

McLoughlin, L. (2020) 2023. *You Look Like Me* Podcast. https://podcasts.apple.com/gb/podcast/you-look-like-me/id1537873411. Accessed November 18, 2023.

Morrissette, M. 2008. *Choosing Single Motherhood: The Thinking Woman's Guide*. New York: Houghton Mifflin Company.

Paplinska's Lucy. 2015. *Sperm Donors Anonymous*. Sensible Films.

Pepperell, J. 1995. *The Posthuman Condition: Consciousness Beyond the Brain*. Bristol: Intellect Books.

Ravitsky, V. 2012. Autonomous Choice and the Right to Know One's Genetic Origins. *Hastings Center Report* 44 (2): 36–37. https://doi.org/10.1002/hast.286. Accessed November 12, 2023.

Rothwell, J. 2010. *Donor Unknown*. Met Film/Redbird.

Sloane, L. 2007. *Knock Yourself Up: A Tell All Guide to Becoming a Single Mom*. New York: Penguin.

Stevens, B. 2001. *Offspring*. FilmRise.

The Donor Conceived Community. 2023. https://donorconceivedcommunity.org/. Accessed November 12, 2023.

The Donor Conception Network. 2023. The Donor Conception Network. https://dcnetwork.org/
———. n.d. Personal Stories. https://dcnetwork.org/useful-info/personal-stories
We Are Donor Conceived. 2023. https://www.wearedonorconceived.com/. Accessed November 18, 2023.
Wolfe, C. 2009. *What Is Posthumanism?* Minneapolis: University of Minnesota Press.

CHAPTER 2

Cyborg Conception: The Solo Mother as a Cyborg Not a Goddess

Abstract Situating the chapter in the 1980s in which goddess ideology and cyborg liberation coincided with the establishment of the Single Mother by Choice community (SMC), I examine how the Solo Mother by Choice (SMBC) can be interpreted as a cyborg mother who combines technology (assisted reproductive technology and gamete donation) and reproductive biology to conceive without a partner. I consider the 'social reality' of the cyborg and argue that the SMBC marks a step away from traditional heteronormative reproduction and nuclear family dynamics to instead represent a binary adjacent family model of one parent from conception.

Keywords Assisted reproduction • Cyborg • Donna Haraway • Donor conception • Family • Fatherlessness • Feminism • Fertility • Gamete donation • Goddess • Mythology • Single mother • Solo mother

REFLECTION

Technology is quite literally beginning to rewire the way we do family. (Smith-Windsor 2005)

In 2018, I stood in a glass lift with four other women ascending London's Shard to the Lister Fertility Clinic. The lift was silent and the five of us stood staring out at the expanding horizon without commenting on the beauty that stretched before us. Somewhere at the top of The Shard, on viewing platforms, tourists were staring at the same view—the sprawling metropolis dotted with tufts of green and embroidered with web-like roads. No doubt, the tourists were excitedly pointing out the twisting Thames and distinctive landmarks like Tower Bridge. We didn't. We said nothing and then sat in the waiting room staring at our feet, avoiding eye contact. I felt such affinity with these faceless, voiceless, nameless women. All I knew about these strangers was that we shared a profound desperation—we all wanted children and, for various reasons, needed help to achieve that.

Like the women with whom I shared a space, I didn't know and couldn't control the workings of my own body. It was my intent, as it had always been since I was old enough to comprehend motherhood, to be a solo parent. So, I found myself sitting in a fertility clinic not because I had fertility issues but because I needed sperm. But, on the train on the way into London it hit me that I actually didn't know anything about my reproductive system—what if it wasn't functioning correctly? What if I had a blocked tube? What if I didn't have any eggs or the ones I had were rubbish? What if, what if, what if? By the time I entered the glass elevator I was on an emotional tightrope that just got higher and higher as we ascended the levels of The Shard. I found myself imagining my womb—something I had never given much thought to before—as a black hole within me. A frightening and incomprehensible space. I didn't understand this void I carried around with me and now it was the most important thing about me.

Before my consultation I had presented the clinic with five vials of blood and was awaiting results of what they called a fertility "MOT" (a fertility check-up)—these results would reveal the mysteries of my body. Did I ovulate? I didn't know. Are women supposed to know? Presumably most women did know about ovulation patterns because the question was on the form I struggled to complete. I also floundered at the question about whether I had struggled to conceive naturally, because I had never tried; I wasn't sure whether to circle yes or no and so wrote a mini essay in the margins. Did I have polycystic ovarian syndrome? No idea. Endometriosis? Presumably not. Had I ever had abdominal surgery (that one was easy): no. In my consultation I become a list of data and none of it I understood. This is me (or, rather, this was me in 2018):

TSH	4.74 mu/L
T3	5.8 pmol/L
T4	9.9 pmol/L
FSH	7.9 iu/L
LH	4.8 iu/L
Estradiol	129 pmol/L
AMH	12.80 pmol/L
Progesterone	28.9
CMV	negative

My data was compared to the data of others and on a chart displayed on my doctor's computer screen I was diagnosed as 'low end of normal with a raised thyroid'.

| Treatment | IUI with donor sperm MOT 20+ and 300 ui injections of Gonal-F and Ovitrelle. |
| Chance of success per round | 15%. |

As I descended in the glass lift, the city welcomed me back into the chaos, but I was transformed. I perceived there to be order now. I felt like a different person to the one who entered the lift an hour before. The desperation that bubbled within me was eased somewhat by the pamphlet in my hand and the medication in my bag. I was comforted by numbers I barely understood and felt bolstered by a drug I hadn't researched. In the year to come I would flood my body with daily doses of 400 micrograms of folic acid, Vitamin D, and "fertility superfoods" like pomegranate, pineapple core and Brazil nuts. When I came to attempt intrauterine insemination (IUI), the stimulant I injected into my stomach stimulated my follicles and the Ovitrelle made me ovulate to schedule; the sperm I ordered was thawed, washed, and inserted into my uterus with a needleless syringe. The whole process I embarked on was subtitled in laymen's terms as "medicated/natural" on my paperwork.

It was an uncomfortable binary because in my mind the medicated aspect rendered the whole process "unnatural"; but the conception itself was natural in the respect that sperm penetrated egg within one of my fallopian tubes. I pondered the naturalness of the process as a nurse called Rachel held my hand while Elena inseminated me with sperm which had been passed through a hatch in the wall by a laboratory technician. Sperm still met egg somewhere in the twisty swamp of my reproductive system just like they would have in the "traditional" way. In *Biological Relatives*, Professor of Sociology Sarah Franklin describes assisted fertilisation as a 'new technology of sex' (2013, 21). I understand that Franklin is referring to the scientific process of reproductive cells merging to create a diploid zygote—that sperm and egg fusion is sex and that IUI (intrauterine insemination) and IVF (in-vitro fertilisation) technologise that primordial act. However, with Rachel's hand in mine, I didn't feel like I was a pioneering consumer of a new technology of sex; I didn't view it as a technology nor as sex. We were making a baby and it involved the introduction of sperm to ovum but at the heart of it all was hope, desire, and love. Was it so different to any other conception?

The IUI was successful and seven months later my babies were born. Unfortunately, they were two months early and were ushered into the Neonatal Intensive Care Unit where they would stay for four weeks. I tried to occupy my mind by learning about the technology of the incubator. I came across the essay 'The Cyborg Mother' by Jaimie Smith-Windsor who, like me, had once sat next to an incubated premature child.[1] She wrote about how the machine takes on the role of mother for premature new-borns. The conclusion of her article questioned the very idea of family in the era of human mechanisation:

> The day I gave birth to a cyborg, I began to understand how every human has become a collaboration of machinic and biological matter. The human condition is mediated by technology. The metanarrative of being cyborg ignores ethical questions. The machine can't ask, What would the world look like without mothers? Or, for that matter, fathers? Technology is quite literally beginning to rewire the way we do family, the way we know humanity. (Smith-Windsor 2005)

Technologies of sex. Technologies of family. In a way they are all talking about the growing dominance of technology and how it can affect the authenticity of the world, the subject, and human action. I don't really know what they mean by the word "technology" when they make such claims: hardware, sociotechnical systems, methodology?

But is it even so radical? When Stephen Kline was debating the inconsistent use of the term 'technology' in 1985, Donna Haraway was unpicking the fabric of what human/nonhuman and natural/technological are in her Cyborg Manifesto. Then, years later Smith-Windsor claims she birthed a cyborg due to the mediation of technology in a biological process. I'm unconvinced that this mediation is actually new at all and that the 'technology' we all nebulously speak of even has definition anymore.

Before I had intrauterine insemination, I underwent a process called a hysteroscopy which is a type of endoscopy to check the uterine cavity for any issues that might prevent "natural" conception through intrauterine insemination. I watched on a screen while the doctor threaded a telescope through my cervix and snaked it around my womb; it had a camera and torch on the end; a dye was inserted, and I watched the blue bloom flood my ovaries and fallopian tubes. I saw a hidden world with alien terrain: pink tunnels with red webs, grey transparent sheets of membrane, and pulsing, beating walls. How, I wondered, could anyone map this geography and understand the primal workings of this deeply buried system?

I didn't understand it in 2018, but the ancient Greeks did way back in the BCEs.[2] They peered into the body aided by candlelight and mirrors; the development of this technique was once termed 'a magic lantern' (Sircus 2003, 124). The gynaecologist tells me this as we voyeuristically gaze into my sapphire-stained womb and see "normal function". The idea of the magic lantern is so poignant to me. The "magic" of being able to intervene in a biological process that deals with cells like the ovum which is a miniscule 0.1 mm; and the symbolism of a lantern that not only hopes to illuminate the mysteries of the womb but to provide a hopeful light for those trying to conceive.

Aren't we all born into technological systems which just gain complexity over the centuries? Smith-Windsor's baby (like mine) was placed into an incubator which is just a more complex version of the prototype developed in the late 1800s. Mediated impregnation—now called fancy terms like intrauterine insemination—builds on the work of John Hunter who used a syringe to impregnate a patient in the 1770s (a technique previously perfected on animals).

We are all cyborg. Everything is a technology when the term is applied so widely.

Family, also, is changing. Smith-Windsor noted this. From the traditional heterosexual nuclear family structure to same sex couples and single parents with their donor-conceived offspring; from family construction via sexual intercourse to mediated impregnation. How we think of family has changed; this isn't a technology nor a product of science—it marks the evolution of society.[3] To me, this is positive.

What we understand family to mean has always been nebulous and changeable. I am reminded again of the Greeks. Families in classical societies—like Ancient Greece—included members beyond the nuclear formation which is why many scholars use the term 'household' instead of family to describe complex kinship connections including the presence of wet nurses.[4] Teresa Morgan describes ancient families as 'a yarn of many strands' (2011, 223). Thinking about this more generally, we might imagine family as rooted in biological connections while the household is an architectural phenomenon. This distinction was made by John Bodel and Saul M. Olyan, who distinguish between genetic connections and the habitat in which people unite (2008, 3). However, to me, contemporary families seem to be increasingly "architectural": constructed through bringing together blood relatives, adopted relatives, donor-conceived relatives, blended families, extended families, communities, and friends. So, yes, a yarn of many strands … from antiquity to now.

Yet, I do agree that there is also something cyborg about the way families are done now, especially for the solo woman who encounters reproduction as a process necessarily mediated by technology. There is also something cyborg about the ways we learn about our bodies today and understand fundamental "natural" processes through data. However, it isn't just the technology that makes conception "cyborg" but the dissolving of the binaries that once traditionally denoted reproduction: man/woman, natural/unnatural, biology/technology, unprocessed/data. The solo mother through gamete donation is the architect of a new way of making families. Smith-Windsor lamented the advent of the Cyborg Mother but, I wonder, what does it really mean to be a cyborg mother?

INTRODUCTION: THE 1980s TRIPARTITE MOTHER: SINGLE, GODDESS, AND CYBORG

In 1985, Donna Haraway concluded her influential essay 'A Cyborg Manifesto' with the line, 'I would rather be a cyborg than a goddess' (1991, 181). Haraway's preference for cyborg existence comes after intense interest in the 1970s and 1980s in goddess feminism. In fact, a year before Haraway's statement, psychiatrist Jean Shinoda Bolen published *Goddesses in Everywoman: A New Psychology of Women* (1984) in which she presented her Jungian-inspired theory that women can identify in their behaviour and psychology the symbolism of ancient Greek goddesses including the Great Mother Demeter. Bolen's work responds to what Jennie Klein identifies as increased attention to goddess worship in the 1970s (2009, 580). Indeed, the goddess was read by some feminists in the 70s and 80s as a push against patriarchal systems (Daly 1973) and a shift towards feminist spirituality (e.g. *WomenSpirit* magazine 1974–1984). However, despite Bolen rejecting the stereotypical reading of women as "acceptable" (maiden, wife, mother) and "unacceptable" (whore and shrew), she still connects women with the idolatry of the goddess and dependency on a "god". Interestingly, in the same decade, Psychotherapist Jane Mattes chose to become a mother without a partner and started the organisation 'Single Mothers by Choice' (SMC) in 1981. SMC is now more commonly known as Solo Mother by Choice (SMBC).

In this chapter, I examine how in the 1980s the SMBC pathway was becoming increasingly popular during a period in which goddess idealism and the cyborg movement were co-existing. Building on from the introductory outline in Chap. 1, this chapter explores more clearly how I am using the term cyborg by examining the development of the cyborg concept over time and across theoretical framings. I will argue that the SMBC signifies the transcendence of reproductive limitations and "goddess" mother stereotypes in both practical and speculative ways. Here I ask, in what ways does the SMBC embrace the cyborg and reject the goddess?

Cyborg and Solo Motherhood by Choice

In the introduction, I spoke in brief about the significance of the cyborg in my reading of the SMBC movement. In this first section, I want to unpack more clearly how the cyborg has developed conceptually since the 1960s. To support my understanding of cyborg conception, I want to look at three ways of defining the cyborg: as an extension of human capability, as a melding of biology and technology, and as an enhancement of the human through technological reliance.

The word 'cyborg' was coined in 1960 in *Astronautics* (developed from the paper 'Drugs, Space and Cybernetics') by Manfred Clynes and Nathan Kline. They write about adapting human bodies as a recommended way to cope with space travel: 'If man attempts partial adaptation to space conditions, instead of insisting on carrying his whole environment along with him, a number of new possibilities appear' (1960, 27). The solution was the cyborg. For Clynes and Kline the cyborg was the realisation of a cybernetic control system: 'The Cyborg deliberately incorporates exogenous components extending the self-regulatory control function of the organism in order to adapt it to new environments' (1960, 27). For Clynes and Kline the cyborg would not be a 'slave to the machine' for the human would adapt to the machine leaving them 'free to explore, to create, to think, and to feel' (1960, 27). Although Clynes and Kline suggested using technology (pharmaceuticals and environmental controls) to enhance the physicality of the human, they did not suggest the incorporation of mechanical components into the body. Neither does the *Oxford English Dictionary*, which defines cyborg as: 'A person whose physical tolerances or capabilities are extended beyond normal human limitations by a machine or other external agency that modifies the body's functioning; an integrated man–machine system' (*OED*, s.v. "cyborg"). This definition refers to cyborg existence as the enhancement of human capabilities by external technology.

However, many scholars view the cyborg as a more intimate fusion of organic and technological matter. The cyborg, for Christine Cornea, represents a 'melding of what were previously seen as separate and divided: the human/machine, the human/nonhuman, the human self/Other' (2008, 275). For Cornea, the cyborg enables us to 'question and contest the premises of what it means to be human' (2008, 287). David Rorvik uses the term 'meld' to describe the cyborg and the 'destruction' and 'construction' involved in hybridisation (1975, 11). The cyborg 'meld' results in a process of 'man-mechanised, machine-humanised' through a fusion of the artificial and organic (Rorvik 1975, 15). Alison Muri defines cyborg as an 'organic machine that is steered or governed by a homeostatic mechanism' (2007, 19). Many definitions work on this principle. These readings present the cyborg as an organic entity enhanced by technology (internally or externally with the body) to extend human ability.

Many scholars who interpret the cyborg as a physical 'meld' of the organic and the technological note that the human becomes cyborg through technological reliance. While Rorvik speaks of the medical cyborg as being prosthetically enhanced (e.g. artificial limbs), he also states that reliance upon the computer makes the human a cyborg through dependence on tools (1975, 13). Similarly, for Andy Clark, the human does not need to be invaded with technology (implants, wires, and microchips) to be cyborg, as the human is programmed and mechanised as part of a new human condition: 'we shall be cyborgs not in the merely superficial sense of combining flesh and wires but in the more profound sense of being human-technology symbionts' (2003, 3). Clark argues that humans rely so heavily on artificial tools that they form part of our living structures (2003, 5–6).

In Haraway's work, her Manifesto combines these understandings of the cyborg and for this reason it is useful to explore it in more detail. Haraway defines her cyborg as 'a cybernetic organism, a hybrid of machine and organism, a creature of social reality as well as a creature of fiction' (1991, 149). The first part of this definition ('hybrid of machine and organism') aligns with the early definitions of the cyborg as a fusion of biology and technology; the second part of the definition I will return to shortly. Often, when the cyborg mother is discussed, she is often described as having biological function assisted by technology in order to conceive and therefore is often conflated with the IVF mother. This is because IVF, as opposed to IUI (which is one of the least invasive of types of mediation), comes with a variety of technological interventions. Whether a partner's sperm or donor sperm is used, the female reproductive system receives the majority of intervention including medicated suppression of the menstrual cycle, medicated stimulation of ovaries, transvaginal ultrasounds to monitor egg maturation, surgical egg collection, and the transference of embryos into the womb via catheter. There are even "add-ons" including endometrial scratching and embryo glue (both are claimed to help implantation), and assisted embryo "hatching".[5] The significant enhancement and manipulation of the body through IVF is well documented in articles like Susi Geiger's 'On Becoming a Cyborg and Paying for It' (2006). Geiger describes the use of IVF technologies to 'make up for any potential "shortcomings" of their own or their partners' all too human constitutions' as a 'cyborgification' (Geiger 2006, n.p.).[6]

Cyborgification, as seen through IVF, does a number of complex things with the human reproductive process including aiding, stopping, starting, and enhancing it. So, in many ways IVF can be seen simultaneously as being part of, helping, and even replacing some human processes within conception. We must also remember that IVF occurs on a spectrum with a "so-called" Natural IVF option which does not use fertility drugs. Natural IVF, despite reading ironically, is discussed unironically as a treatment option by clinics such as Assisted Reproduction and Gynaecology Centre (ARGC) and CREATE. As Tine Ravn explains in *Lived Realities of Solo Motherhood, Donor Conception and Medically Assisted Reproduction* (2021), medically assisted reproduction presents 'puzzling paradoxes' through 'imitating and destabilising "natural" forms of procreation and kinship relations in diversifying hitherto unquestioned binaries, such as nature/culture, biology/sociality, and sex/procreation' (n.p.). The paradoxes exposed by Ravn are similar to the cyborg contradictions and realities expressed by Haraway. Ravn leans on Haraway, most notably her 1992 essay 'The Promises of Monsters' in which Haraway articulates a fusion between 'bodies and technology and its influence on our under-standings of gender and identity'; Ravn explains that 'the use of assisted reproductive technologies serves as precisely such a fusion, one which dis-rupts the nature/culture distinction to alter our understanding both of how we are made and of 'natural categories such as family and kin' (2021). Understanding the influence of assisted reproductive technologies is to appreciate that we are not only discussing the extremity of medically assisted reproduction through IUI and IVF, but how, as Ravn notes, 'we live in a biotechnological culture in which bodies and technologies become increasingly intertwined' (2021). As I stated in the introduction, even "natural" conception can be presented as mediated: ovulation tracking apps, fertility supplements, fertility acupuncture, and digital pregnancy tests. Pregnancy is negotiated through scans, blood tests, dopplers, and so on. In an infertility study by Helen Allan (2007) she found that patients perceived technology to be immensely reassuring, more so than the advice of human consultants: 'These practices [ultrasound] reinforced infertile women's beliefs that medical technology could provide an explanation of infertility and control fertility.'[7]

In my reflection at the start of this chapter, I described how I felt that I had become a collection of data-based signifiers. As a patient I had become a collection of hormone levels, scans, and blood tests. The way in which I was to understand my body and journey towards motherhood was narrated—almost exclusively—by value-laden facts obtained through technological intervention, whether this was through biochemical analysis in a laboratory or through hysterosalpingo-contrast sonography. When my biodata was compared with my peer group, tweaks were made to my biology in an attempt to yield better data results. My follicle-stimulating hormone (FSH) was 7.9; Gonal-F (300 ui) was administered to stimulate the follicles for better conception odds. My consultant understood when it was a good time to attempt IUI because the data readings were at their most ideal. It was a balancing act—increase AMH, lower FSH, lower thy-roid, increase endometrial thickness and so on. When I did successfully conceive, I conceived twins; this was not a massive surprise to my clinic because it was understood statistically that patients had a 30% greater chance of a multiple pregnancy following pregnancy success through Gonal-F. Paradoxically, my twins were "naturally" conceived as they were IUI babies and not IVF babies (fertilisation occurred within my body)[8] but "unnatural" because medication forced my body to release more eggs than normal.

As I explained in the introduction, where Robbie Davis-Floyd and Joseph Dumit (1998) argue that babies are *born* cyborgs, I suggest that they are *conceived* as cyborgs. Before we even get to conception, we see a "cyborgification" in how the body is read as data and how diet, exercise, pharmaceuticals and surgery can improve these data values. To be a cyborg we do not need to embed chips and wires into our bodies; to be cyborg, as Clark (2003) argues, we just need to be significantly influenced by technology and this influence can be seen in the very ways in which we view the body as a data source and then use this information to enhance the chance and potential to conceive. While this happens for all conceiving people and couples to various extents, the SMBC can be said to profoundly engage all definitions of the cyborg. For the SMBC, fertility treatment extends the capabilities of the body; interventions like freezing donor gametes [9] and IVF demonstrate a melding of biological and technological processes; and the use of aids like ovulation trackers and the capacity to read the body as data suggest technological reliance to some extent.

Yet, despite the numerous benefits of this technology to solo patients, assisted reproduction is often articulated as being for couples. In Sarah Franklin's *Biological Relatives* (2013), which draws on Haraway's work, IVF is described as popularised by the 'narratives and hopes of couples seeking children' (31–2). When Franklin claims that 'after IVF we had a new kind of biological kinship with technology', this symbiosis was more accessible to heterosexual couples (many of whom do not require donor gametes) (2013, 32).[10] Franklin states that '[i]n vitro fertilization exists because mere biology is not enough' (2013, 32), but for many SMBC, biological infertility is not what propels them to access IVF/IUI: instead, "social infertility" is the issue (this will be explained later). Biology, in this case, is often enough, but technology (including donated gametes) is employed to fill a gap rather than replace a function. The cyborg then, is not an end of traditional ideas of conception and biology, but rather represents additional opportunities afforded to the human through biomedical collaboration. However, any sort of melding is a problem for anti-cyborg thinkers such as Mary Harrington who worry that cyborg-like tech and organic collaboration will distance humans from their inherent natures. For me, human evolution is cyborg evolution—different names for the same changing and developing over time. As humans evolved so did their use of tools until we arrived at today when human and tools have opportunities for profound collaboration. For some, like Harrington, this is concerning (in similar ways to concerns over large technological shifts, such as the printing press, the loom etc.); but for others, like me, it marks an opportunity for human action that was desired but difficult—if not impossible—before. Contrary to concerns articulated by Harrington, traditional ideas do not cease to exist—heterosexual intercourse and sexual reproduction are not at risk; they continue to represent the statistical "norm". The "norm" is not under pressure, but there is new space for alternative pathways. When Harrington writes that human nature is at risk of 'liquefaction' (2023, 79), I instead identify complication. The cyborg does not suggest a dilution of the human, it opens up new ways of being and this chimes with the second part of Haraway's definition.

In the second part of her definition, Haraway describes the cyborg as 'a creature of social reality as well as a creature of fiction' and it is the ways in which the SMBC is narrated in contemporary culture that is of interest here (1991, 149). While I am not proposing that the SMBC pathway be read through the lens of Haraway and her specific understanding of the cyborg, there are many points on which Haraway's work can be used to help us think about how solo parenthood through gamete donation challenges resistive binaries surrounding traditional ideas of the family and reproduction. For example, when Haraway writes, 'The boundary between the physical and the non-physical is very imprecise for us' (1991, 153), this is true for the SMBC as someone who has physically conceived a child through the fusion of male and female gametes but also presents a 'non-physical' reality in which the resulting child is not of two parents but of one. There is an important distinction between gamete provider and father; to have a fatherless child may seem an oxymoron but, as Adam Bostic notes, 'The cyborg is nothing if not a mass of contradictions both real and imagined' (Bostic 1998, 358). Haraway's cyborg helps articulate how the SMBC bypasses the limitations of heteronormative framings in reproduction discourse. While Haraway argues that 'cyborgs have more to do with regeneration and are suspicious of the reproductive matrix and of most birthing' (1991, 181), I argue that the SMBC destabilises this 'matrix' by "regenerating" (making new) how conception can occur and be communicated.[11]

Haraway and I part ways quite dramatically on the issue of reproduction. I, a mother to biological children and an academic scholar on reproduction, stand in opposition to Haraway's later works in which she argues that we should focus on kinship, not baby making. For Haraway, the cyborg represents regeneration rather than reproduction and should pose a solution, of sorts, to planetary problems—for example, overpopulation.[12] In Haraway's understanding, "Cyborgs for Earthly Survival" becomes linked to "Make Kin Not Babies" (2015, 161).[13] I do not want to delve into this too much as this book is not about Haraway, but instead about how, what I term "cyborg conception" can help us unravel oppressive and resistive traditional narratives on reproduction and family building. In essence, my thinking on cyborg conception is to suggest that the cyborg is about regenerating what reproduction is and how it is done and what families it can produce. In this respect, just as the SMBC is a 'deviation from convention' (Roberts 2019), I deviate from Haraway.

In highlighting the coexistence of Haraway, Bolen, and Mattes in the 1980s during the start of the SMBC's movement into more mainstream treatment and public understanding, I am highlighting how a push against dualistic thinking, the dawn of new reproductive technologies, and more radical understandings of family construction had synchronicity (although not harmony). This leads me to wonder how the idea of the cyborg (as a hypothetical and literal construct—which has existed in science and philosophy pre and post Haraway) can provide the tools and language to identify in the SMBC something quite radical.

There might be an instinctual rejection of the term "cyborg" or a suspicion of its application in its suggestion of SMBC as somehow abnormal, monstrous, or unnatural. This is not what I intend to convey. Think of cyborg as an abbreviation for "boundary breaker" and it becomes less jarring. The cyborg—for me—is three things: mediated by technology in some way, influenced by certain scientific and technological advancements even if only environmentally, and a philosophical concept in which traditional boundaries fall under scrutiny. This understanding has been shaped by research—since the 1960s—on the cyborg as the ability to be 'free to explore' (Clynes and Kline 1960); as extending human limitations (OED, s.v. "cyborg"); as the hybridisation of organic and technological (Cornea 2008, Rorvik 1975, Muri 2007); as the influence of an increasingly technological society (Clark 2003; Davis-Floyd and Dumit 1998); and as 'a creature of social reality' who is paradoxical through challenging established binaries such natural/unnatural (Haraway 1991, 149). When I define cyborg conception I refer to an intentional application of technology (from DIY home insemination kits through to IVF) to mediate and assist the biological act of reproduction; specifically here, the use of donor gametes and the establishment of a paradoxical single parent family from conception is cyborgic in the respect that sexual reproduction and dual-parenting "norms" are disrupted.[14] Cyborg conception enables women to procreate when ordinarily this would not be a possibility (for a variety of reasons). It is liberational in the respect that it creates opportunities for women to solo parent when, historically, single parenting has been viewed with significant criticism. By repositioning solo parenting as involving intent, decisions, and choices there are opportunities to destigmatise the "victimised" single mother.[15] The SMBC can be seen as an example of a turn in post 80s society towards a complete rethinking of family construction. Although Haraway and I disagree on many elements of the cyborg, we find agreement in terms of how the cyborg represents freedom from restrictive binary understandings of self. This is why, like Haraway, I would 'rather be a cyborg than a goddess' (1991, 181).

GODDESS AND SINGLE MOTHER

What, though, is meant by the goddess, and specifically for this discussion on the cyborg mother, what is meant by the goddess-mother? Returning to Jean Bolen, writing at the same time Haraway was pondering the cyborg, she speaks of empowering women through helping them discover the goddess within: 'When she knows which "goddesses" are dominant forces within her, a woman acquires self-knowledge' (1984, 5). Bolen presents us with different types of mothering (Artemis, the mother whose children do not fulfil her; Athena who longs for her children to gain independence; Hera who prioritises her spouse over her children; the detachment of Hestia; the inconsistency of Aphrodite; and the insecure struggling mother Persephone); but positioning Demeter as 'the Great Mother' establishes an ideal mothering style (1984, 22). Demeter is described as 'the most nurturing of the goddesses', a woman who 'may also not be able to say no to getting pregnant' and experiences a 'compelling force toward getting pregnant' (Bolen 1984, 171, 189, 172–3). In Bolen's work, the single or solo mother is not discussed (despite the prevalence of single mothering in Greek mythology). If, as Bolen suggests, 'Many Demeters marry young' and this 'may fit with a girl's own Demeter proclivities to have a family rather than an education or a job', then the successful mother goddess is interpreted as conceiving within the nuclear family model (1984, 179).

The unsuccessful Demeter goddess mother can be read as the "unfortunate" childless woman or the single/solo mother who is pregnant in circumstances 'far from ideal' (Bolen 1984, 189). Traditionally, the single mother has been presented as a problematic figure in society linked to dysfunctional child-rearing environments as identified by Gideon Calder, who notes that it is often understood that '[t]he children of single parents are more likely to live in poverty, and less likely to do well at school' (2018, 421). As Ross Parke notes in *Future Families*, often single mothers are viewed stereotypically negatively: 'The public perception of single mothers as poor, impulsive, irresponsible, and unfit for parenthood is widespread. Many assume that they are an economic drain on the state and collect welfare to survive' (Parke 2013, 68). However, this is not only a contemporary concern. As Jane Juffer notes in her historic overview of the treatment of single mothers, an unwed mother with an illegitimate child was considered 'ruined' and suffered hellish treatment ('hell hath no punishment like the treatment people give a "fallen woman"' (2006, 12)).

Single mothering has traditionally been viewed as "accidental", "lamentable", and as something that has circumstantially happened without choice. Indeed, why would a woman choose to be a single mother when it is so demonised? In a chapter entitled 'What Is Wrong with Technology?' Naomi Cahn notes that developments like IVF cause social controversies, one of which is the capacity for single people to intentionally produce children as solo parents; this, she notes, has led critics to view reproductive technologies as directly undermining matrimony (2009, 165). While single fathers have been historically imagined as "put upon" and "heroic" for child rearing upon the untimely and inconvenient absence of a mother/wife (either because she died or proved "unreliable"), the single mother has been presented as a problematic issue for religion, society, culture, and the economy. In the 1960s, Carole Anderson spoke about the stigma associated with being a single mother, noting that 'they told us we would be ruining our children's lives by keeping them'. She further comments that single mothers were told that by raising their children solo their children 'would be ridiculed at school as bastards, or grow up to be homosexual because they lacked a father image, or would live in poverty forever because no decent man would marry us' (cited in Corea 1985, 47). Single mothers routinely found themselves unable to keep or gain employment, expelled from their place of education, and unable to source childcare meaning that, for many single mothers, 'few of us had any option but to surrender our children' (Anderson cited in Corea 1985, 47). Writing in the 1990s, Ruth Sidel notes that single mothers were viewed as responsi-ble for many of the problems within American society, from high crime rate and addiction to poor educational outcomes and poverty (1996, 4). Describing single mothers as often demonised as the "enemy within", Sidel reflects that historically mother-only families were considered to be "dangerous" and an "underclass" with single mothers viewed as "virtually irredeemable, lazy, dependent" (Sidel 1996, 1).[16]

Historically, single motherhood caused specific cultural and social problems for offspring as fatherlessness and father absence affected inheri-tance and social status. The demonisation of the single mother is an his-toric issue referenced in texts since antiquity. For example, in the Homeric Hymn to Apollo in which Olympian King and Queen Zeus and Hera compete to create offspring solo, Zeus produces the wise and beautiful Athena but Hera produces Hephaestus who is described as monstrous. As Daniel Ogden argues in his article on fatherlessness in ancient Greece, the message here is that a 'mother can only produce misshapen monsters on their own' (2009, 117). There are also numerous references to the mon-strousness of single motherhood and the threat the single mother poses to married couples. One such example can be seen in the Jewish legend of Lilith, the first wife of Adam who refused to submit to her husband and left Eden. Alicia Ostriker notes that 'Lilith attempts to seduce men, and that she slips between a man and his wife to steal drops of his semen and make demons from it to plague mankind'. Ostriker also mentions that '[t]raditional households' sought to protect themselves from Lilith (1993, 91).[17] It is possible here to see how the SMBC can be read as connected to the demonised Lilith—a "difficult" independent woman who is resis-tant to marriage, the procurer of sperm, the creator of illegitimate chil-dren, and a woman who poses a risk to the traditional nuclear family ideal.

In anti-donation debate, negativity about single parent families is often rooted in the prioritisation of the nuclear family as articulated by David J. Velleman (see Velleman 2015) and Professor Sidney Callahan, the latter of whom argues, 'Cultural norms, based on reason and natural evolution, have mandated the unity of genetic, gestational, and rearing parents. A mated and committed pair-bonded couple exists in an acknowledged extended biological kinship system' (1998, 92). With the demonisation of women reproducing outside the 'pair-bonded' dynamic comes a gendered concern in which women are actively encouraged not to exercise control of their reproductive function. Ultimately the message is the same as it was back in the myth of Hera and Hephaestus: a solo mother family is abhorrent.

During feminism's 'Second Wave' (roughly covering the 1960s–1980s) the stigma of single motherhood started decreasing—especially after 1970 (Vandenberg-Daves 2014, 251). For example, landmark developments like the Guardianship Act 1973 amended the law of England and Wales to make 'the rights of a mother equal with those of a father' (1973, 1) and in doing so reimagined women and men as on equal footing in terms of parental rights. The 1970s introduced rights for maternity leave, repercussions for sexual harassment and tried to ensure workplace equality between the sexes. The British Women's Liberation Movement championed legislation for equal treatment and this included reproductive rights. As Florence Binard states, this movement occurred during, and was influenced by, 'diverse contestation movements that had emerged in the 1960s in Britain, parts of Europe and also in the United States' (2017). In America, greater support for women's rights (including reproductive rights, for example, *Griswold v. Connecticut* in 1965 and *Roe v. Wade* in 1973), the championing of women in power (National Women's Political Caucus, founded in 1971), and advancements made to equal treatment with men (Equal Pay Act, 1963—the UK followed suit in 1970[18]) meant that women were enjoying greater freedoms and opportunities. Although there remained extensive issues relating to fair pay and treatment of women, these freedoms would not only underpin the Third Wave (1990s–) but lay the foundational groundwork to support SMBC in our contemporary.[19] Mikki Morrissette in her memoir as a SMBC notes that 'the pioneers of Choice Motherhood grew up feeling better able to create their own destinies than previous generations of women did' (2008, xviii). Likewise, Jane Juffer notes that the efforts of the LGBTQ+ movement and feminist movements opened up 'new possibilities for mothering without men' due to the increasing independence of women (such as career opportunities) and an opening up of what family can mean beyond the nuclear formation (2006, 4). In a sociological research study conducted by Linda Layne, she found that 'American women who purposely undertake motherhood without the involvement of a male partner tend to be beneficiaries of second-wave feminist achievements in the areas of expanded educational and employment opportunities' (2014, 1). In another study, Layne found that most SMBC were highly educated, older mothers with a degree of financial stability (2015, 1155). Ravn notes that SMBC are often understood to be 'financially independent, well-educated, middle to upper-class women in their late thirties and forties with well paid jobs and supportive social networks of family and friends' (2021). I do think this profile has changed with the growing interest in "DIY"/informal/unregulated donor conception which, due to lack of industry price-tag running into the tens of thousands, means that women of all backgrounds and circumstances can pursue SMBC through known donation.

This is not to say that reproductive freedom has been achieved. The overturning of *Roe v. Wade* (1973) on June 24, 2022 by the US Supreme Court legally rules that abortion in the United States is not a constitutional right. The ramifications of this ruling mean that women cannot seek pregnancy termination in the way they wish in many US states: individuals must either travel (at cost) to a location in which abortion is legal or gestate and birth a child against their will—a ruling which disproportionally impacts single women. We must wonder, and be vigilant, about other freedoms that could fall under pressure next (will emergency contraception be restricted or banned in law and policy?) and if freedoms will be restricted in the UK as well as in the US (we must not underestimate transatlantic influence). Although these questions are primarily playing out in America, it is of global concern; as we witness the unravelling of protections established in the 1970s, will we see other reproductive rights erode? Will fertility treatment, IVF specifically, become restricted due to the creation and banking of embryos?[20] Will we see renewed restrictions of fertility treatment to unwed people and same sex couples? It is ironic that, in the US, SMBC represents a step forward for women to choose solo conception but the same woman is stripped of the right to choose not to gestate an unwanted pregnancy. Abortion is beyond the scope of this book, but it is worth remembering at this juncture that reproductive rights are neither universal nor stable. It is also worth highlighting the hypocrisy here for solo parents: that banning abortion will force the creation of demonised non-traditional families—such as single mother families; yet SMBC are also demonised for choosing to create non-traditional families. Whether a solo parent by choice or by circumstance both types of parenting appear on a "spectrum of selfishness" in which a woman is criticised for both unplanned and planned pregnancies.

Both abortion (choosing not to gestate) and solo motherhood through gamete donation (choosing to gestate) are viewed by some as extreme feminist acts leading to condemnation in some circles and the rescindment of certain reproductive rights. In terms of SMBC, Gill Rye suggests that 'any women who choose to conceive without men are commonly positioned as a threat to the good functioning of the social order' (2010, 232). Indeed, it is precisely the threat to rigid social order that the cyborg represents; the choice to become a solo parent is an act that reclaims bodily freedom and permits the reimagining of the body and person as a cyborg. The cyborg and goddess are not dichotomies; the cyborg consumes the goddess/god and gendered binaries and is instead an identity-fluid hybrid. The cyborg's irony disrupts the illusion of the goddess and challenges the ideal the goddess embodies. The SMBC dislocates the fallen woman/goddess dichotomy that has oppressed women since ancient times and offers conception without men, mothering without a partner, and solo reproduction as both reality and fiction.

Yet, even for SMBC supporters, there is a tendency to compare the SMBC to the nuclear family ideal and to suggest that solo parenting is a contingency that mourns a co-parenting relationship. Susanna Graham argues that SMBC do not pose a threat to the nuclear family model but instead are 'reworking their ideas about motherhood and relationships in an aim to salvage at least some of the nuclear ideal they had imagined for themselves' (2012, 97). Contrary to Graham's analysis, I suggest that the SMBC is not trying to salvage 'some of the nuclear ideal' but instead represent a new type of family formation that exists beyond the binary parameters that mark heteronormative parenting structures. The one-parent offspring of the SMBC reflects the social and imagined reality of solo parentage even if this contradicts biological reality. While, for Haraway, we are all cyborgs ('we are all chimeras'), for me the SMBC at their most ironic (conceiving solo) is an ultimate example of cyborg conception by refusing 'seductions to organic wholeness' (1991, 150).

CONCLUSION

In 1991, Haraway's 'Manifesto' was republished in *Simians, Cyborgs and Women*. Just two years later, the Donor Conception Network charity was formed to support donor-assisted families. In the same decade, Mattes published her handbook *Single Mothers by Choice* (1997 [1994]) to help prospective solo mothers consider gamete donation for family creation. If the 1980s can be called a decade in which the single mother was identified as mourning her inability to achieve a 'normal family' (Quinn and Allen 1989), the 1990s could be described as a decade in which the solo mother by choice (SMBC) tried to unabashedly rearticulate solo parent families as a legitimate form of family planning.

Haraway argues: 'By the late twentieth century, our time, a mythic time, we are all chimeras, theorized and fabricated hybrids of machine and organism' (1991, 150). She is not alone in imagining the cyborg as something that has happened to us all through hybridisation. Although N. Katherine Hayles estimates that '10 percent of the U.S. population are cyborgs' due to the application of prosthetic enhancement or replacement (such as pacemakers), she states that *all* humans are cyborg through hybridisation with regard to gender, politics, and other cultural realities (1990, 277). Everyone is cyborg, then. Even "feminist against progress" Mary Harrington—who is extremely concerned about the cyborg and its argued dystopian potential—notes that she too, for better or worse, is 'very much a creature of the cyborg era. I'm permanently welded to the internet. I got my job through Twitter, I'm a fully paid-up cyborg' (Harrington and Allen 2022). However, when I speak of a "cyborg conception", I am thinking not only of the technicalities of the cyborg and the saturation of technology within contemporary western society. I am also imaging how the SMBC marks a step away from traditional heteronormative reproduction and nuclear family dynamics to represent a binary adjacent family model of one parent from conception.

At the start of this introduction, I reflected on 'The Cyborg Mother' essay by Jaimie Smith-Windsor in which she concluded, 'Technology is quite literally beginning to rewire the way we do family' (Smith-Windsor 2005). Is this true? I have given this statement a lot of thought while writing this chapter. I was born in the 1980s and was raised within a caring and supportive nuclear family unit. My devoted parents instilled in me the importance of love and family and are, unsurprisingly, very supportive of my choice to become a SMBC. I was born in a decade of notable feminist and technological shift; throughout my developmental years I saw the changing landscape of LGBTQ+ rights and more positive visibility. I was sixteen at the turn of the century and the internet complemented my teen years with wider opportunities for connection and, in turn, new communities. By the time I made my decision to become a SMBC in 2018, I felt embedded in a much richer tapestry of identity, family, and community. By choosing to become a SMBC I was not rejecting the nuclear unit that was so beautifully demonstrated to me through the stable and committed marriage of my parents, I was instead enjoying the opportunities for a different type of family. One that was just as stable and loving as my parents'. These opportunities were enabled through shifts in societal attitudes towards tolerance, respect and celebration of non-traditional ways of understanding gender, identity, family, and parenting. Technology has simply helped the actualisation of these new understandings. Technology is not the catalyst of change here—change comes from people. So, is technology itself rewiring family?

No, I thought, *technology is not rewiring how we do family, family is rewiring the way we do reproduction.*

NOTES

1. Interestingly, Mary Harrington notes that the idea for her "anti-cyborg" book came from her experiences of motherhood, specifically that she did not feel separate from her child (2023, 3). I, too, started to think about the thematic content of my book during the early days of motherhood but precisely because I was separated from my babies and was trying to understand the mediation of technology. While Smith-Windsor—like Harrington—would see technology as a threat, I saw salvation and hope. Harrington and I have a lot in common—both English Literature graduates, both mothers, and both scholars writing on cyborg reproduction, but it is on that last point—about the benefits and perils of cyborg reproduction—we fundamentally disagree.
2. I refer to Greek history throughout to chime with Jean Bolen's focus on Greek goddesses.
3. While there is an evolution of family, it is worth noting—as the rest of this book will illustrate—that the nuclear family is still very much presented as the norm by which the other family constructions are judged.
4. I do not wish to overlook the hierarchies present here and do not suggest that the ancient household was unproblematic or that household members were treated fairly or equally. My point is that the designation of family is not historically stable.
5. "Add-ons" are, and should be, under scrutiny. There is limited evidence to suggest that they are effective. The HFEA has a rating system for add-ons and the ones mentioned here have limited evidence of directly securing treatment success (pregnancy).
6. This tendency to align cyborg mothering with technological intervention bleeds into experiences of the Newborn Intensive Care Unit (NICU) which has been described by Jaimie Smith-Windsor as mediated cyborg mothering (2005).
7. Although reassuring, as Ravn notes, the saturation and 'naturalization' of a spectrum of technology within conception pathways can pose a problem for feminists 'since these technologies on one hand may help defeat involuntary childlessness, which causes many women great distress but on the

other hand, they may add to the reproduction and essentializing of gender expectations to reproduction, which can intensify the distress of infertility' (2021).

8. Although as stated earlier, some IVF is called Mild or Natural IVF.

9. Even the brokerage of sperm renders the gamete technologised in a sense. A sperm bank stock is not representative of the donor but is instead reframed as a number, a motility factor, and a value (example, Donor 1111, Mot: 40, £1450).

10. Of course, the medical system will prioritise the largest patient group (heterosexual couples).

11. I personally believe it is possible to be suspicious of the reproductive matrix and its oppressive structures while not rejecting reproduction.

12. I will unpack this claim about regeneration briefly—Haraway reflects on the salamander which has regenerative healing abilities and says that 'we require regeneration, not rebirth' (1991, 181). On reading Haraway's idea of regeneration, Denise Handlarski explains that '[f]or some women, the idea of cyborgean regeneration frees women from the imperative of biological reproduction' which has been long articulated as a goal in some feminist discourse because 'Women being reduced to their biology has, in any location, been a site of female oppression' (2010, 78). A quick response is to perhaps argue that reproductive freedom, reproductive technologies, and choice motherhood challenge ideas of oppression, but not in the way in which Haraway is discussing the cyborg or the importance of regeneration and kinship. Haraway is suspicious of reproduction in all its forms—not just biological sexual reproduction but the reproduction of structures, politics, patriarchy, and so forth. Handlarski sums it up nicely when she writes that 'Haraway's blasphemous text that calls for regeneration to replace reproduction enacts its criticism of grand narratives'. (2010, 90).

13. Although Haraway prefers the idea of replication to reproduction and is more interested in kinship than biological bond, Haraway also states that '[t]he inalienable personal "right" [...] to birth or not to birth a new baby is not in question for me; coercion is wrong at every imaginable level in this matter' (2015, 164).

14. I am focusing primarily on the UK regulated sperm donor conception industry with reference to the US. Obviously, the idea of the cyborg and the idea of reproductive freedom is different and under pressure depending on geographic location and the influencing factors of religion, politics, culture, and industry.

15. This book does not intend to offer an historical overview of the single mother, but rather identify how influential stigmatisation has been.

16. As well as class connotations, these stereotypes can also take on racist connotations.

17. Jean Renvoize (2023) notes that '[w]omen have been traditionally blamed for almost everything from the beginning', citing the myths of Pandora to Eve.
18. There was already a long history of pay-related and gender-fairness related protest. For example: in 1888, 200 women took strike action against Bryant & May due to poor and unfair working conditions; this is commonly known as The Match Girl's Strike (see Francis-Devine and Ferguson 2020).
19. Obviously, the feminist waves and the establishment of movements and Government issued Acts have not eradicated problems. For example, in the UK despite the Equal Pay Act the 'UK's overall median gender pay gap is still 17.3%' (Francis-Devine and Ferguson 2020).
20. As this book was being prepared for publication in February 2024, Alabama Supreme Court ruled that embryos have rights as 'extrauterine children'. This judgement impacts treatment like IVF, which deals with the creation of, storage of, and sometimes destruction of embryos. In response many clinics in Alabama have paused IVF treatment.

References

Allan, H. 2007. Experiences of Infertility: Liminality and the Role of the Fertility Clinic. *Nursing Inquiry*. 14(2): 132–139. https://doi.org/10.1111/j.1440-1800.2007.00362.x. Accessed July 16, 2023.

Binard, F. 2017. The British Women's Liberation Movement in the 1970s: Redefining the Personal and the Political. *Revue Française de Civilisation Britannique.* http://journals.openedition.org/rfcb/1688. Accessed May 8, 2023.

Bodel, J., and S.M. Olyan. 2008. Introduction. In *Household and Family Religion in Antiquity*, ed. John Bodel and Saul M. Olyan, 1–4. Oxford: Blackwell.

Bolen, J.S. 1984. *Goddesses in Everywoman: A New Psychology of Women*. New York: HarperPerennial.

Bostic, A.I. 1998. Automata: Seeing Cyborg through the Eyes of Popular Culture, Computer-Generated Imagery, and Contemporary Theory. *Leonardo* 31(5): 357–361. https://www.jstor.org/stable/1576595. Accessed April 24, 2022.

Cahn, N.R. 2009. *Test Tube Families. Why the Fertility Market Needs Legal Regulation.* New York: New York University Press.

Calder, G. 2018. Social Justice, Single Parents and Their Children. In *The Triple Bind of Single-parent Families: Resources, Employment and Policies to Improve Wellbeing*, ed. R. Nieuwenhuis and L.C. Maldonado, 421–436. Bristol University Press.

Callahan, S. 1998. The Ethical Challenge of the New Reproductive Technology. In *Health Care Ethics: Critical Issues for the 21st Century*, ed. J.F. Monagle and D.C. Thomasma. Gaithersburg: Aspen Publishers.

Clark, A. 2003. *Natural-Born Cyborgs. Minds, Technologies, and the Future of Human Intelligence*. Oxford: Oxford University Press.

Clynes, M.E., and N.S. Kline. 1960. Cyborgs and Space. *Astronautics*, September 26–76. 75–76.

Corea, G. 1985. *The Mother Machine: Reproductive Technologies from Artificial Insemination to Artificial Wombs*. Cambridge: Harper and Row.

Cornea, C. 2008. Figurations of the Cyborg in Contemporary Science Fiction Novels and Film. In *A Companion to Science Fiction*, ed. David Seed, 275–289. Oxford: Blackwell.

Daly, M. 1973. *Beyond God the Father: Toward a Philosophy of Women's Liberation*. Boston: Beacon Press.

Davis-Floyd, R., and J. Dumit. 1998. *Cyborg Babies: From Techno-Sex to Techno-Tots*. London: Routledge.

Francis-Devine, B., and D. Ferguson. 2020. 50 Years of the Equal Pay Act. *House of Commons Library*. https://commonslibrary.parliament.uk/50-years-of-the-equal-pay-act/#:~:text=On%2029%20May%201970%2C%2050,pay%20gap%20is%20still%2017.3%25. Accessed November 13, 2023.

Franklin, S. 2013. *Biological Relatives. IVF, Stem Cells, and the Future of Kinship*. London: Duke University Press.

Geiger, S. 2006. On Becoming a Cyborg and Paying for It: Invocations of Motherhood in the IVF Industry. *Advertising & Society Review* 7 (3). https://doi.org/10.1353/asr.2007.0004. Accessed November 12, 2023.

Graham, S. 2012. Choosing Single Motherhood? Single Women Negotiating the Nuclear Family Ideal. In *Families—Beyond the Nuclear Ideal*, ed. Daniela Cutas and Sarah Chan, 97–109. London: Bloomsbury Academic.

Guardianship Act. 1973, c29. https://www.legislation.gov.uk/ukpga/1973/29/enacted. Accessed December 12, 2023.

Handlarski, D. 2010. Pro-creation—Haraway's 'Regeneration' And the Postcolonial Cyborg Body. *Women's Studies* 39: 73–99.

Haraway, D. 1991. A Cyborg Manifesto: Science, Technology, and Socialist-Feminism in the Late Twentieth Century. In *Simians, Cyborgs, and Women: The Reinvention of the Nature*, 149–182. New York: Routledge.

———. 2015. Anthropocene, Capitalocene, Plantationocene, Chthulucene: Making Kin. *Environmental Humanities* 6: 159–165.

Harrington, M. 2023. *Feminism Against Progress*. Croydon: Forum.

Harrington, M., and Allen, E. 2022. Cyborg Feminism. *Public Discourse*, December 8. https://www.thepublicdiscourse.com/2022/12/86306/. Accessed January 30, 2024.

Hayles, N.K. 1990. *Chaos Bound: Orderly Disorder in Contemporary Literature and Science*. London: Cornell University Press.

Juffer, J. 2006. *Single Mother: The Emergence of the Domestic Individual*. London: New York University Press.

Klein, J. 2009. Goddess: Feminist Art and Spirituality in the 1970s. *Feminist Studies* 35(3): 575–602. http://www.jstor.com/stable/40608393. Accessed January 5, 2021.

Kline, S.J. 1985. What Is Technology. *Bulletin of Science Technology & Society* 1 (215): 215–218. http://bst.sagepub.com/content/5/3/215.citation. Accessed December 7, 2022.

Layne, L.L. 2014. A Changing Landscape of Intimacy: The Case of a Single Mother by Choice. *Sociological Research Online* 20: 1–16.

———. 2015. I Have a Fear of Really Screwing It Up: The Fears, Doubts, Anxieties, and Judgments of One American Single Mother by Choice. *Journal of Family Issues* 36: 1154–1170.

Mattes, J. 1997 [1994]. *Single Mothers by Choice: A Guidebook for Single Women Who Are Considering or Have Chosen Motherhood.* New York: Three Rivers Press.

Morgan, T. 2011. Ethos: The Socialization of Children in Education and Beyond. In *A Companion to Families in the Greek and Roman Worlds*, ed. Beryl Rawson, 217–230. Chichester: Blackwell.

Morrissette, M. 2008. *Choosing Single Motherhood: The Thinking Woman's Guide.* New York: Houghton Mifflin Company.

Muri, A. 2007. *The Enlightenment Cyborg. A History of Communications and Control in the Human Machine 1660–1830.* London: University of Toronto Press.

OED (Oxford English Dictionary Online). n.d. s.v. cyborg, n. Accessed June 12, 2023.

Ogden, D. 2009. Bastardy and Fatherlessness in Ancient Greece. In *Growing Up Fatherless in Antiquity*, ed. S.R. Hubner and D.M. Ratzan, 105–119. Cambridge: Cambridge University Press.

Ostriker, A. 1993. *Feminist Revision and the Bible.* Cambridge: Blackwell.

Parke, R.D. 2013. *Future Families: Diverse Forms, Rich Possibilities.* Oxford: John Wiley & Sons.

Quinn, P., and K.R. Allen. 1989. Facing Challenges and Making Compromises: How Single Mothers Endure. *Family Relations* 38(4): 390–395. https://www.jstor.org/stable/585743. Accessed December 4, 2023.

Ravn, T. 2021. *Lived Realities Of Solo Motherhood, Donor Conception And Medically Assisted Reproduction.* Emerald Studies in Reproduction, Culture and Society.

Renvoize, J. 2023. *Going Solo: Single Mothers by Choice.* London: Routledge.

Roberts, G. 2019. *Going Solo: My Choice to Become a Single Mother Using a Donor.* London: Piatkus.

Rorvik, D. 1975. *As Man Becomes Machine.* London: Abacus.

Rye, G. 2010. Lesbian Mothering in Contemporary French Literature. In *Textual Mothers/Maternal Texts: Motherhood in Contemporary Women's Literatures*, ed. Andrea O'Reilly. Waterloo, ON: Wilfrid Laurier University Press.

Sidel, R. 1996. *Keeping Women and Children Last: America's War on the Poor.* New York: Penguin.

Sircus, W. 2003. Milestones In The Evolution Of Endoscopy: A Short History. *J R Coll Physicians Edinb* 33: 124–134. http://www.rcpe.ac.uk/journal/issue/journal_33_2/8_milestones_in_endoscopy.pdf. Accessed March 4, 2023.

Smith-Windsor, J. 2005. The Cyborg Mother. *Radical Philosophy* 129.

Vandenberg-Daves, J. 2014. *Modern Motherhood: An American History.* New Brunswick: Rutgers University Press.

Velleman, J.D. 2015. Family History. In *Beyond Price: Essays on Birth and Death,* 1st ed., 61–78. Cambridge: Open Book Publishers. http://www.jstor.org/stable/j.ctt17w8gwg.7. Accessed March 4, 2023.

CHAPTER 3

Liminal Experience: The Solo Mother, Fertility Clinics, and Ambiguous Loss

Abstract In this chapter, I focus on how the Solo Mother by Choice (SMBC) is represented in anti-donation discourse and in fertility clinics. Despite research evidencing that donor-conceived children are not disadvantaged, anti-donation debate focuses on the moral ambiguity of creating single parents. Although most UK clinics welcome solo patients, most fertility clinics focus on couples, biological infertility, and pregnancy loss and therefore, because SMBC often do not fit these narratives, they are sometimes overlooked and under-represented. These experiences can lead to feelings of liminality in which SMBC exist in an ambiguous space between ethical/unethical, fertility/infertile, advantaged/disadvantaged, and natural/unnatural.

Keywords Anti-donation • Assisted reproduction • Bioethics • Cyborg • Disadvantage • Donna Haraway • Family • Fatherlessness • Fertility • Fertility clinics • Fiction • Gamete donation • Grief • Goddess • Liminality • Loss • Moral philosophy • Mythology • Selfishness • Single mother • Solo mother

G. Halden, *Cyborg Conception*, https://doi.org/10.1007/978-3-031-59386-4_3

REFLECTION

[M]edicalisation does not resolve these liminal dimensions; it tolerates the ambiguity and uncertainty while at the same time contributes to the creation of ambiguity and uncertainty. (Allan, 2007)

When I returned from maternity leave, I re-entered life as a university lecturer in modern and contemporary literature and culture. I was asked to deliver a class on assisted reproduction and its representation in contemporary literature. I chose to talk about Mieko Kawakami's fiction novel *Breasts and Eggs* (2020), which follows the journey of Natsuko Natsume, a single woman who decides to conceive solo through sperm donation. I started my lecture with a quote from Natsuko's friend Rika: 'If you want a kid, there's no need to get wrapped up in a man's desire [...] There's no need to involve women's desire, either. There's no need to get physical' (Kawakami 2020, 320). When I first read the book during the confinement of newborn parenting, I was moved by that line. I remember humming my agreement and underlining the sentence with a pencil while rocking my twins in little bouncy chairs with my feet.

Natsuko's pathway was more fraught than mine; living in Japan where fertility treatment for solo women is illegal, Natsuko needed to be more resourceful and far braver than me. Over the course of the novel, I became attached to her—this bold and determined woman. *Breasts and Eggs* was also the only novel I had read that represented the reality of solo motherhood neutrally and covered the various issues with this pathway such as known and anonymous donations. I was excited to share this book and Natsuko's journey with the postgraduate class I had been assigned.

During the lecture, I spoke about new attitudes towards family planning and the ways in which technology has facilitated diverse family formations. I spoke about the importance of storytelling our origins and how instrumental storytelling is for establishing identity and encouraging inclusion of non-nuclear family types within society. I introduced Kawakami's novel as an expression of these issues.

In the seminar after the lecture, the class divided into pairs and I gave them a series of questions to consider. I wandered around the room enjoying the lively debates at each desk and came to stand near a pair who had been assigned question five:

5. How are marriage and heterosexuality presented in the text?

I never have an answer in mind when I set a question because I'm interested more in the discussion and debate. However, I suppose I expected students to reflect on Natsuko's friends who represent different relationship dynamics. Along with the questions, I had given students an extract pack including a scene in which Natsuko is at lunch with a group of old work friends discussing the conditions under which they would save the life of their husbands—a scene which reveals that many of the group are unhappily married or married for social stability. Rather than focusing on this scene, my students were discussing the "unhealthy-ness" of donor conception; one student, I'll call her Lizzie, had heard that children born to single parents were statistically more likely to be impoverished and turn to crime. The point was made that even though Natsuko might have been unhappy in a relationship, it would have been preferable to conceive and raise a child within one.

I intervened and clarified that extensive research shows that children born to solo parents via donation thrive and, when compared to offspring born within a nuclear family, are not disadvantaged emotionally or psychologically. I quoted Professor Susan Golombok, who said it better when she wrote succinctly but effectively: 'Children do just as well in "new family structures" as in the traditional family' (Golombok 2015b).

Susan is somewhat of an academic celebrity in the SMBC community, having published a wealth of positive research on donor conception. I actually met Susan at a conference where she was presenting on the findings of her longitudinal study of families assisted by surrogacy. She related that over the twenty years her team had been gathering data that showed that, whether born from egg, sperm, or embryo donation or via surrogacy, children and adolescents did not present as being disadvantaged by having one biological parent when compared to offspring born via 'natural conception'.[1] I attended the conference while my university was on strike. I snuck into the conference feeling like a traitor, but I was there for a very specific reason. Not to see Susan, but to listen to a panel discussion led by children who were in some way connected to surrogacy—some were donor-conceived. I wanted to hear what they had to say. I had read plenty and I had heard Susan's presentation, but I wanted to sit in a room with donor-conceived children and hear their stories. Two of the panel were twins and I found myself drawn to them and their words as if they were somehow more valid to me than any other. It was a positive encounter. Raised with awareness of their conception story, these children spoke confidently about being donor-conceived and expressed no unrest about how they came to be in their family unit. This comforted me then and still does now.

I told Lizzie about the panel, but the student remained convinced that donor conception is selfish. Lizzie asked me, not knowing that I am a SMBC, why a single woman would want a biological child to raise alone? I said nothing, not wanting to prejudice a class so I instead asked the student to think about Natsuko's motivation. Lizzie concluded that Natsuko was selfish. I suppose Lizzie is right to some extent—Natsuko chose to have a baby because she wanted one and prioritised that want above all other things, including Japanese law. However, is Natsuko alone in reproductive selfishness? An observation by SMBC Mikki Morrissette stuck in my mind: no-one asks married people why they want a biological child; their motivations remain unquestioned (2008, 8). So instead, I asked, 'Should only heterosexual couples have biological children?'

Lizzie thought about it for a moment and then made a conclusive statement that wanting and pursuing biological children is completely selfish; she threw her hands up in the air and said something that made us all laugh, me included: 'Adopt don't shop.'

That evening I sat on the train mulling 'Adopt don't shop' over in my mind. The day before on Twitter (as it was known back then) the app told me 'I might like' tweets from the CEO of @adopteefutures. I clicked to have a look and the latest anti-adoption tweet concluded, 'The entitlement to another person's child is wild'. I spent a good hour working through that account, reading the many anti-adoption and pro-guardianship debates. While looping around the Circle Line on the Tube, I was reminded of Christine Overall's book *Why Have Children?: The Ethical Debate* (2012)—I had read it years ago on the same train bound for Tower Hill. Specifically, Overall's conclusion stuck with me: limiting procreation itself is important in the era of 'procreative carelessness' (2012, 176).

What did this all mean?

Don't shop.
Don't adopt.
Don't procreate.

If Natsuko was selfish, wasn't everyone else? The only conclusion I think anyone can reach in these ethical debates is that the dominant notion seems to be that heterosexual couples are naturally entitled to produce a single biological child through intercourse and raise it; everyone else is obligated neither to birth nor rear children.

Is family really so stacked in the favour of married heterosexual couples?

INTRODUCTION: THE LIMINAL SPACE BETWEEN NATURAL AND UNNATURAL

Robbie Davis-Floyd and Joseph Dumit in *Cyborg Babies* identify that (during their time of writing in the late 1990s) most people readily accept 'natural conception through sexual intercourse as the norm and artificial conception as the anomaly' (1998, 6). I argue that artificial conception should not be viewed as an anomaly and believe that by thinking about "artificial reproduction" only in the extremes of IVF (for example) we miss the casualisation of every day reproductive assistance. Davis-Floyd and Dumit separate the artificial from the natural when they contrast 'invasive, often painful' procedures (such as IVF) with 'more organic or holistic' options for fertility which are 'rendered invisible' (1998, 7). I do not believe that "procedures" should be separated from the organic; the cyborg represents a large spectrum between organic and artificial rather than a harsh divide. As noted previously, even the "organic" route can be a pathway of bodily enhancement, manipulation, augmentation, and refinery. Choosing, for example, to dramatically increase fruit intake in response to research suggesting that a fruit heavy diet can prevent miscarriage is a strategic intervention for reproductive success: a way to steer what Davis-Floyd and Dumit call the 'body-machine.' When Davis-Floyd and Dumit argue that we are in a 'technomania' in which reproductive assistance (extended also to birthing assistance) has 'naturalized technobirth', I do not accept this as a problem; when they argue that 'it has become unnatural to give birth at home' I argue that in certain situations it is inadvisable to birth at home (in my case my babies needing NICU care would have died) (1998, 9). I gave birth without pain medication nor intervention (no forceps, for example)—was this a natural birth but in an unnaturalised hospital environment? Are these distinctions helpful?

I believe that they are not and instead argue that birthing has evolved as the birthing environment and birthing tools have evolved. It was once "natural" for one in three women to die in childbirth; our ability to improve environment and tools has increased life expectancy for mother and child. Forceps are not "posthuman" tools of the modern cyborg but instead ancient tools of early birthing dating back to the sixteenth century. Is "natural" therefore the absence of any intervention? Why is natural presented as always "good"? I am reminded of the execution of Euphemia Maclean in 1591 who, among other "crimes of witchcraft", was accused of not birthing "naturally" because she accepted pain relief during labour. Having survived childbirth, Maclean was then burned alive for her "unnatural crimes."

Many women across the globe conceive and birth without any intervention or mediation: they conceive through sexual intercourse, they do not change their habits (they do not change diet, take supplements, or alter working patterns), they then freebirth without intervention or assistance. This can be viewed as natural; but it does not need to be framed as the antithesis of the cyborg or as better. Today it is common for vaginal birth to be described as "natural birth" in contrast to caesarean birth; the vaginal birth is positioned as "natural" even if assisted with an epidural, suction, and forceps. The cyborg is the adaptation of the human to the environment and technology—all of which inform the other. The mother who has undergone assisted reproduction and assisted birthing is not unnatural in her cyborg environment but only in contrast to how "natural" is understood outside this space.

In this chapter I explore how the SMBC can be viewed as "unnatural" in contrast to the "natural" traditional nuclear family structure which is often framed as "normal" and "advantaged." SMBC, whom I argue represent a profound and systemic realisation of the cyborg through both a melding with technology and representing a new social reality of reproduction, end up existing in a problematic liminal space in which they are welcomed to access treatment but within clinics that are not always designed for single patients because pregnancy, as many anti-donation thinkers argue, (should) happen as part of "natural" relations within marriage. This in turn impacts how SMBC experience fertility treatment and navigate the complexity of grief and loss as part of their journey to try and conceive a baby.

So far, I have shown how the cyborg has been presented as a binary breaking, boundary resisting entity and we have understood this to be a largely positive and liberational development, especially for solo women. The cyborg, especially in Donna Haraway's understanding, is connected to liminality because it represents transition and intermediacy—the cyborg is the occupation of a space between distinct states/ideas/things. However, in this chapter I complicate what it means to be 'in between' fixed conditions by looking at problematic ways in which the SMBC is shunned and overlooked as they fall into a murky liminal space in ethical debate and clinical treatments that rely, to various degrees, on the familiarity and "normality" of the heterosexual couple. In the latter part of the chapter, I also consider the ambiguity of loss for SMBC who might grieve "natural" conception.

Obligation Not to Conceive: SMBC and Anti-donation Discourse

To start, I want to first look at how the SMBC is discussed in anti-donation debate. In the last chapter, I noted that one of the reasons SMBC fall under scrutiny is because there remains stigma surrounding the moral ambiguity of creating single parents who are stereotypically presented as a problematic presence within society. This stigma has been shaped by historical treatment of single women who were actively encouraged not to parent solo (Vandenberg-Daves 2014, 112–114). In more contemporary contexts, it speaks volumes that academic collections like *Mama PhD* (a collection of over forty essays on mothers pursuing PhDs while childbearing/rearing edited by Elrena Evans and Caroline Grant 2008) and *Motherhood, the Elephant in the Laboratory* (a collection of over thirty essays by mothers in academia edited by Emily Monosson 2008) do not include single mothers. Both *Mama PhD* and *Motherhood, the Elephant in the Laboratory* inadvertently work to separate the realm of academia from the single mother who is more commonly associated in mainstream culture with a lack of education and means. Even in academic texts that discuss the 'single mother' these women are often presented as reckless people who have negligently reproduced: Professor Browne C. Lewis in *Papa's Baby: Paternity and Artificial Insemination* reflects, 'My older sister is a free spirit. She does not let much bother her. She dances to her own beat. When I was almost a teenager, my sister left home to find herself, and returned home expecting her first child. There was no mention of the baby's father. During my niece's formative years, she was raised by my parents' (2012, 7). In Judith Solomon and Carol George's study on how upbringing impacts mothering, the only single mother case study is of Sara, who is 'chaotic', 'angry', 'out-of-control', 'helpless', and 'frightened' (2006, 283–4).

Collectively, these observations chime with moral philosopher David J. Velleman's claim that donor conception produces 'disadvantaged' children.[2] In his article 'Family History' (originally published in 2005), Velleman argues that donor conception is unethical and suggests that donor-conceived people are 'handicapped' due to being raised without knowing both biological parents (2015a, 74). The publication of 'Family History' joined a range of work from other philosophers in the early 2000s who also argued against donor conception and prioritised the nuclear family as an ideal (see Browning 2003, 2007; Almond 2006; Austin 2007). Margaret Somerville (2011), who draws on Velleman's 'Family History', extends Velleman's claims and suggests that donor-conceived people suffer as a result of being donor-conceived and therefore suggests that donor conception is against the Hippocratic Oath. However, contemporary scholars such as Susan Golombok (2015a, 2015b), Amanda Roth (2016), Ross D. Parke (2013), and Ezio Di Nucci (2016) argue that anti-donation arguments refer to outdated models, outdated research, and historic cases of unregulated donor conception which are now against industry recommendations in the UK and the US (more on this later).[3]

Velleman first refers to the 'disadvantaged child' when he writes, 'Much as we love disadvantaged children, we rightly believe that people should not deliberately create children who they already know will be disadvantaged' (2015a, 67). For Velleman, the donor-conceived person is 'disadvantaged' because they do not know their biological roots:

> In my view, people who create children by donor conception already know—or already should know—that their children will be disadvantaged by the lack of a basic good on which most people rely in their pursuit of self-knowledge and identity formation. In coming to know and define themselves, most people rely on their acquaintance with people who are like them by virtue of being their biological relatives. (2015a, 67)

Velleman argues that children should be raised by both biological parents as identity is shaped by genetics, nurtured by biological relatives, and shaped through ancestral resemblance. So strong is this conviction that Velleman associates birthing donor-conceived children with wilfully causing birth defects:

> [T]he fact that a child would be glad to have been born cannot justify us in conceiving it. Congenitally handicapped people live rich and fulfilling lives

into which they are glad to have been born, but a woman who is taking a teratogenic medication has an obligation not to conceive a child until she has stopped taking it. (2015a, 73–4)

Velleman is not merely arguing that a woman should not jeopardise the health of her foetus (which is something many people would agree with); he is suggesting that to reduce 'suffering' women should not birth 'disadvantaged' people. This view suggests a eugenical perspective prejudiced in favour of heteronormative (and able-bodied) supremacy. Consequently, whether by choice or by circumstance, it is, according to Velleman, impossible to justify planning a family when both biological parents will not be involved in the raising of that individual. Moreover, there is an obligation for certain people not to conceive a child unless they can follow the heteronormative, co-parenting norm.

In shaping his argument about the importance of child-rearing by both biological parents, Velleman reflects on how instrumental ancestral knowledge is for his own negotiation of self. He writes, 'For information about my appearance, they [ancestors] may not be as good a source as an ordinary mirror; but for information about what I am like as a person, they are the closest thing to a mirror that I can find' (2015a, 70). This is a privileged perspective that assumes all children borne to heterosexual couples will be furnished with ancestral knowledge when many may not know their extended families.[4] Furthermore, this perspective suggests biological scripting which is only helpful if one's ancestors were positive role models, as no-one looks to their grandparents to explain why they might be lazy or liars. Nevertheless, nostalgically reminiscing about idyllic heteronormative upbringing when presenting anti-donation arguments is not unique to Velleman. Lewis reflects on her fortune compared to the 'disadvantaged child' of a single mother: 'Growing up, I was the only one of my friends who had a father living inside the home. As a result, we were the only family on our street with a telephone and an automobile' (Lewis 2012, 7). Here, Lewis reflects on the "problem" of the single parent family. In this case the "problem" is linked to economic disadvantage, which is common. As Anna Furse notes, 'single mothers have become the bêtes noires of the Welfare State' (2001, 239). Writing in 2001, Furse notes that due to concerns over the disadvantages single parenthood could bring, many fertility clinics displayed negative attitudes to treating single women with many clinics claiming that they would refuse treatment (2001, 239).

It was only in 2008 that UK law changed and allowed clinics to treat solo women without prejudice. Before 2008, clinics were expected to first assess whether the resulting child would be disadvantaged if raised without a father before offering treatment to SMBC. The 1990 legislation read: 'A woman shall not be provided with treatment services unless account has been taken of the welfare of any child who may be born as a result of the treatment (including the need of that child for a father), and of any other child who may be affected by the birth' (Human Fertilisation and Embryology Authority 1990, c37). Since the legislative change in 2008, same-sex couples and solo women have been able to access fertility assistance without the assumption that these reproductive pathways are inherently problematic. Yet, despite growing numbers of SMBC and 'greater acceptance' of solo parenting through gamete donation, Morrissette notes that SMBC 'still feel the bite from those who feel they are wrong to bring a child into a fatherless world" (Morrissette 2008, 60). Concerns include stigma that children raised by single mothers will have decreased chances of economic, educational, and societal success. Mary Harrington goes as far as to suggest that without a "good man" a woman cannot successfully raise a child: 'a world where every baby can be welcomed without a loss to women's personhood is self-evidently impossible unless it's also filled with good husbands and fathers' (2023a, 205). Stigma also surrounds the solo parent who is not only described as "selfish" by scholars like Velleman but as abnormal by theorists like Linda L. Layne who describes SMBC as 'maverick moms' who are often associated with the "'uncanny", "creepy", "freaky" and "strange'" (2013, 140). Layne leans on Sigmund Freud's term 'Uncanny' to describe how 'SMCs [single mothers by choice] and lesbian moms engage in a number of practices that traffic back and forth between the familiar and the bizarre, the comfortable and the strange' (2013, 144).

While Christine Overall in *Why Have Children?: The Ethical Debate* notes, 'The choice to procreate is not regarded as needing any thought or justification' (2012, 2), this is not the case for SMBC whom, it seems, exist in a liminal space in which they are invited to access fertility treatment but are constantly faced with having to defend their choice to procreate. Heteronormative families are rarely challenged on their right to have biological children even if using donor gametes. The stigmatisation of solo parent families as inherently selfish and abnormal contributes to the general argument that some women 'cannot justify' (to use Velleman's words) conception. There is a gendered concern here in which women are actively encouraged not to exercise control of their reproductive function.

Often judgement aimed at single women concerns the perception that these women either cannot meet or keep a man who is imagined would be an ideal father. As Katherine Mack notes, there is an assumption of what ideal fathering looks like, which is usually 'white, cisgender, heterosexual, and gainfully employed' (Mack 2020, 291). Furthermore, there is the assumption that all fathers must be good fathers—and the presence of a genetic provider is more important than family stability and safety. When Velleman argues that 'the serviceability of single parenting cannot justify the creation of children with the intention that they grow up without fathers of any kind', what is meant by 'father of any kind'? (2015a, 75 fn10). Many children have father figures of a kind: uncles, a godfather, a grandfather, all of whom provide plenty of XY representation.[5] If the "natural" (biological) father is paramount then do we welcome the abusive father, the absent father, the negligent father, the irresponsible father, the imprisoned father? (And, what about the dead father?).

In *Test Tube Families*, Professor of Law, Naomi Cahn, notes that while 'the two-parent model generally is beneficial for children, forcing all families into that model does not benefit children' (2009, 169). There are circumstances in which Velleman accepts different family forms but only when strictly necessary. Velleman argues that when disruption occurs through events like death or divorce, then 'a child is entitled to be raised by parental figures who love it' (2015a, 72). So, he agrees to compromise. Yet, if compromise is deemed necessary when the "ideal" family configuration is disrupted then surely SMBC marks another type of "compromise", in this case *before* conception.[6] Although I will come to memoir in Chap. 5, I am reminded of the words of solo mother Genevieve Roberts who discussed the importance of compromise in conversation with SMBC life coach Mel Johnson:

> I really felt like I would want something based on some sort of security. Not as much as for me but as much for the child. I think it's really important for a child. And there's so much evidence now that security is so important to children [...] I had been burnt by a relationship where I had chosen to divorce. I felt a bit burnt by the relationship where someone had left so swiftly. I really wanted to get it right. Also, I remember one of my friends saying to me, 'You've waited this long, don't settle now.' (Roberts in Johnson 2020)

In many respects, the SMBC can represent a healthy response to conception and child-rearing that bypasses traumas that can be associated with attempting to have a biological child in an environmentally challenging situation even though, technically, it would adhere to a social norm. The SMBC does not have to remain in an unhappy co-habiting model to have a child: 'others, coming of age in a divorce culture, saw Choice Motherhood as a positive alternative to putting a child through the traumas of an unstable marriage' (Morrissette 2008, xviii). As Morrisette notes, with high divorce rates in the UK and US the odds of single motherhood by circumstance are high (2008, 65). Indeed, as Linda Layne reflects, by choosing to become a SMBC disruption is avoided: 'becoming a SMC [single mother by choice] may spare one the risk of an unhappy marriage, divorce, and child custody battle' (2015, 1167).

The stigma of 'disadvantage' due to a family model not reflecting heteronormative co-parenting models not only works to criticise the solo mother by choice (and same-sex couples) but also to undermine and demonise sperm donors as contributors to a societal problem. This demonisation is linked to the "unnaturalness" and commodification of selling gametes and the view that gametes have become "things" to be harvested and used in a technologised process. Matthew Schmidt and Lisa Jean Moore talk of *technosemen* as the product offered by sperm banks—*technosemen* meaning the cyborgification of semen and the way it is viewed as part of a manufacturing process. While I do not disagree that the donation of gametes for donor conception is cyborg, I believe the way '*technosemen*' is described is negatively loaded. Schmidt and Moore describe 'technosemen' as 'the "new and improved" bodily product' in which the "improved" element refers to the testing, diagnosis and analysis of semen (1998, 25). In terms of marketing, Schmidt and Moore suggest that "*technosemen*" is desirable in the market due to being presented as superior: 'fertile, uncontaminated, and genetically "engineered" for desirable traits' (1998, 27). While semen for donor conception is marketed based on accentuating desirable traits, this is not much different to the ways in which people regularly filter potential partners based on likes, dislikes, interests, education, career, family connections, and appearance. In terms of dating apps, the process of "selection" when choosing a potential romantic mate based on listed 'selling points' is not dissimilar to selecting a sperm donor for procreation from a profile. In my case, I chose someone who sounded kind and someone with a background in the Arts (like me). Of course, the major difference is the matter of monetarising gamete donation; however, in the UK, donors are not paid and therefore altruistic donations are more commonplace. The issue of the monetisation of gametes is complicated. Although this sort of cyborg intervention exists within a capitalist model in which the gamete banks and clinics are profiting industries, the donor and recipient have a very different relationship. The donor does not receive a fee and the recipient does not pay the donor. Instead, the recipient pays for the mediatory service of the bank and clinic.[7] The relationship between the donor and recipient is not transactional at all. Furthermore, in many cases, money is not exchanged at all when a known donor is used for home DIY insemination.

In more extreme narratives about sperm donation, the donor is presented as some sort of deviant. Lewis, in her book on artificial insemination, uses the term 'sperm donor' for what she terms the 'fornicating man.' The term fornicating man is already problematic as it paints unmarried but sexually active men as immoral but, additionally, connecting fornication with sperm donation weaponises donation as a slur and consequently links donor-conceived people with antiquated ideas of illegitimacy and shame. Lewis is not the only scholar to connect donor conception with "unnatural" and illicit acts. Professor Sidney Callahan compares assisted reproduction to prostitution (2013). In a similar vein, Mary Harrington speaks of the good father and husband in contrast to the cyborg-era which has created 'sperm donors' which are linked with 'porn-addled pick-up artists, passive-aggressive "male feminists" or bitter, proletarianized male labourers doing grunt work by day and seething online at night' (2023a, 205). There has long been a connection articulated between sperm donation and "seedy" behaviour—often an association made comically. For example, published one year after the birth of the first IVF baby in 1978 was Roald Dahl's *My Uncle Oswald* (1979)—a sex comedy revolving around sperm theft. High-profile men, such as noted artists, are unknowingly being used for the procurement of sperm to be sold illegally to women desperate for 'high quality' gametes. The medical rape of the men is seemingly excused as the men, presented as "fornicating", are penned as deserving of such treatment as a consequence of being sexually active outside monogamy.

When Lewis states that a 'fornicating man' is a sperm donor by having 'donated his sperm by having sex with the woman' she misses the financial, legal, ethical, and altruistic differences between promiscuity (which might accidentally result in conception) and someone who consciously and morally chooses to assist family formation through donating gametes (and thereby severing all legal and ethical responsibility for a resulting child). This is an issue Susanna Graham fails to address in her article for *Anthropology & Medicine* when she distinguishes single mothers through divorce and single mothers through donation based on attitudes towards the absent father. Graham notes a donor can be construed as 'a "truly absent father"': not only physically absent but also little, if any, information about him' (2018, 255). Velleman also contrasts the donor with adoption to highlight a perceived inadequacy of gamete donation: 'we tolerate a practice equivalent to creating a child for adoption. Those who "donate" their sperm and eggs play their role in conceiving children whom they have no intention of parenting' (Velleman 2015c, 106). However, the difference, in these examples, is intent—the intent of the "fornicating" man, the intent of the divorcee, and the intent of a parent placing their child for adoption is extremely different to the intent of a sperm donor. By contrasting sperm donors with men who sire "legitimate" offspring, a wider point is made about societal attitudes to father absence which, here, seems linked to excessive sexual appetite, transactional attitudes towards sex, and an aversion to reproductive responsibility. Velleman, Lewis and Callahan present sperm donors as absconding when there is another type of liminality evidenced here that they miss: sperm donors are not absent fathers because they are not fathers in a social sense at all. More precisely sperm donors do not suggest father absence—in which a fatherly role was expected and then rejected—they are genetic providers who contractually were never going to occupy a fatherly position.

Clarity that donors are not fathers (in a social sense) is significant. There is much to be said about the importance of transparency for donor-conceived people; the UK model which ensures that children born after 2005 can discover identifying information about their donor helps, in some way, with issues of estrangement. Research as well as testimony from donor-conceived people show that it is best for donor-conceived children to be raised with awareness of their donor conception and with the ability to ascertain the donor's identity.[8] I agree with Velleman that it is important to enable offspring to learn their genetic history (known and ID release donation can achieve this); however, when Velleman speaks of a procreative 'standard of adequacy' he is speaking not necessarily about genetic awareness but of nuclear family preference (2015c, 108). Yet, being raised in a heterosexual co-parenting dynamic does not always mean a healthy, stable, or "adequate" environment.

Velleman is not alone in his anti-donation beliefs. Callahan compares the creation of donor-conceived people by infertile couples, same sex couples and solo parents as akin to 'breeding dogs and horses'—something that should not be attempted for humans existing within 'complex familial ecological systems' (1998, 85). This perspective furthers the stereotype that solo parenthood (by chance or by choice) is an inferior type of family formation. The stigmas forwarded by individuals like Callahan actively harm donor-conceived people and donor-assisted families and encourage invisibility of positive representation. The emergence of diverse family structures is not a threat to the traditional family but part of an evolution. Callahan, by referring to cultural norms as shaped by 'natural evolution' and 'reason', misses that cultural norms evolve, as they have done now to include the 'modern' family. Callahan (as well as Velleman) also misunderstands that the statistical norm does not equate to an ideal. Likewise, when Harrington writes that 'heterosexuality is still the default' this does not mean that the default is the best model (Harrington 2023a, 22–3). Harrington states that '[m]ost of us want children; most want a life lived in common, usually with a member of the opposite sex' but, obviously, 'most' means that there is a percentage of people who are not included here (Harrington 2023a, 22–3). This "remainder" should not be dismissed or overlooked because they are not the majority "norm".

The modern family is different from how it was viewed pre-1978 (before the birth of the first IVF baby) when family was defined as a 'cultural unit which contains a husband and a wife who are mother and father of their child or children' (Schneider, 1968). In fact, research has shown that today most people believe that a family is formed by the presence of a child regardless of the formation (for example, solo parenting) (Cahn 2013). The law also recognises new family formations through how "parent" is defined diversely in the law (biological parent, legal guardian etc.). Therefore, new family formations should not be dismissed as inferior. As popular as the nuclear family dream is, it is neither ideal nor reflective of societal trends; on this point The Ethics Committee of the American Society for Reproductive Medicine notes:

> A family traditionally consisted of a man, married to a woman, and their children. The father was the provider, and the mother stayed at home to raise coitally conceived children. This idealized concept never was fully realized and has changed markedly in recent years as a result of high divorce and out-of-wedlock birth rates, adoption, assisted reproduction, recognition of

women's rights, the gay rights movement, the legalization of same-sex marriage in some jurisdictions, and other social and economic factors. (2013, 1524)

In *Going Solo*, Jean Renvoize points out that what constitutes a family has changed in modern times: 'family life as we know it is a new creation of the last two centuries, and contraception, modern medicine and social changes have reduced it to a pale shadow of what it had become by Victorian times' (2023, n.p.). For, as Renoize remarks, the very idea of what family is and what kinship entails has always been in flux and is widely open to interpretation today: 'you don't need a marriage to make a family, you don't need two parents to make a family—you need a common interest of space and money and resources to share. A commune can become a family' (2023, n.p.).

Yet for philosophers like Velleman, 'this new ideology' of family is what anti-donation debate is pushing against (Velleman 2015a, 75). Velleman's preoccupation with the 'selfishness' of donor-assisted procreators suggests that selflessness resides with heterosexual couples who bear children. Therefore, it is often argued that the selfishness of SMBC is rooted in the egocentric want for self-gratification (companionship, the experience of parenting, creating biological offspring etc.): 'the self-interested assertion of will' (Velleman 2015b, 1). And yet, these reasons are not different to the reasons a married couple would give for procreation. Surely any attempt at reproduction could be construed as selfish (certainly in terms of the environmental ramifications of having a child).[9] If the recommendation is to birth one child per person (so two per couple), anything over that could also be considered 'selfish'. As Overall argues, 'those who choose procreation who happen to be single or in a same-sex relationship have no higher burden of justification, I argue, than do those who are married and in a heterosexual relationship' (2012, 137). So, when Velleman declares that 'the fact that a child would be glad to have been born cannot justify us in conceiving it' I argue that, yes, knowing a child would be glad to be born does justify conceiving them because if this is not the case then we wade into the quagmire of "no-one should have children" (Velleman 2015a, 73–74). Ideals (or 'adequacy') are unattainable, impractical, unfeasible, and open up absolutely every configuration of parenting model to criticism. The conclusion such deliberations take us to is an extreme one: ideally, no-one should procreate.

It is suggested that one way the SMBC can sidestep judgement of 'bad mother' is by adopting[10] (Velleman 2015a, 75). But why is it not morally preferable that heterosexual couples adopt instead of procreate? Why did Velleman procreate when he could have adopted an 'alienated' and 'disadvantaged' child? Because judging by Velleman's argument heterosexual couples are viewed as *entitled* to procreate while the rest of society is *forced* to consider alternatives. Consequently, reproduction is reserved for a select few who have chosen to "naturally" have children despite the selfishness of this decision in the grand scheme of the planet. It is in the "naturalness" of sexual reproduction (ideally within marriage) that selfishness of procreation is somehow avoided.

In Morrissette's memoir and guide, she asks whether the prospective SMBC (the reader) has the 'proper motivation' to take on solo motherhood by choice. She attempts to help the reader ascertain their own suitability by asking them a series of questions:

Do I have stability in my life (financial, familial, emotional, supportive)?
Do I have realistic expectations about motherhood?
Have I considered health issues in becoming pregnant?
Can I be flexible and roll with the punches?
If something happened to me, who would take over?
(Morrissette 2008, 12)

These questions are applicable to couples considering having children and any woman considering pregnancy but there seems to be a burden of proof for SMBC who need to prove their capacity to parent (for example economic and social capacity) to counteract accusations of selfishness. However, as Morrissette argues, 'many Choice Mothers agree that giving up time, money, freedom, and an independent lifestyle to raise another human being is not a selfish act' (2008, 65). But even if it is selfish, then it is one selfish choice in an endless list of selfish choices for, as Renvoize states in *Going Solo*, 'whatever they [SMBC] do they will probably be accused of being selfish', whether this is having children with assistance or not having them at all (2023, n.p.).

The decision to parent solo through gamete donation is not only a decision that involves practicalities but one that demands nuanced thinking about the complexities of genetic and nongenetic relationships. Tine Ravn notes, 'Embarking upon solo motherhood entails conscious reflections about how family and kin are to be defined, but we must also regard the decision to become a solo mother as one that is shaped in the complex processes that interlink chosen life plans with available life chances and options' (2021). Becoming a SMBC is not quick, easy, or straightforward.[11] Susanna Graham (2018) argues that SMBC are 'moral pioneers' who 'grapple with the meaning of incorporating donor sperm into their journey to motherhood' (2018, 252). For Graham the moral pioneering manifests when the SMBC must reconcile the belief that she will be a good parent with the unknown element of sperm donation and the impact it will have on her offspring (2018, 261).

In 2023, psychological outcomes for donor-conceived offspring raised with awareness of their origins are not so unknown. In fact, there is a plethora of research being conducted on children born through donor conception. Susan Golombok et al.'s paper published in *Developmental Psychology* (2017), which references Velleman's work, notes:

> Despite the concern that children born through reproductive donation would be at risk for psychological difficulties at adolescence, the findings of the present phase of this longitudinal study of families formed through egg donation, donor insemination, and surrogacy showed that these families did not differ from natural conception families when the children reached age 14.

Golombok concludes, 'Children born through reproductive donation are, by necessity, planned and there is evidence to show that planned pregnancies are associated with more positive psychological outcomes for mothers and children' (Golombok et al. 2017, 1973–4). Golombok is not alone in challenging anti-donation rhetoric associated with moral philosophers like Velleman. Amanda Roth questions the validity of Velleman's anti-donation position in light of evidence proving that 'the very children he presumes to be disadvantaged and raised in inferior families do just as well (or better) than those raised in traditional heterosexual families?' (2016, 42). Likewise, Parke argues in *Future Families* that non-traditional families thrive even though they do not reflect the "ideal" nuclear form (2013, 73). Golombok's research, and the work of Parke and Roth, highlight that instead of promoting the nuclear family as the ideal family formation, any family structure which centralises love and stability is an aspirational family model.

Despite positive regulatory changes in the UK permitting the treatment of solo women without prejudice, dominant anti-donation discourses seem to argue that—law aside—unpartnered women have an obligation not to conceive. Juffer reflects on the numerous freedoms single mothering encompasses including sexual freedom and parenting freedom but rightly asks: 'How free are most single mothers to pursue these possibilities? Some of that freedom is impeded by the privileges that marriage continues to confer' (2006, 10–11). The impediment is often practical—there are financial and logistical advantages to being partnered; however, the impediment is also one of social pressure in which donor conception is framed as unethical. Although asked in 2006, just before legislative changes to make the process more 'freeing', Juffer's question is still pertinent today—how free are women to choose this stigmatised and expensive pathway?[12] Moreover, how welcomed are they?

LIMINAL EXPERIENCE: FERTILITY CLINICS

So far, I have mapped the tricky terrain of anti donation discourse which suggests that "natural" reproduction is preferable to assisted reproduction. I have shown that SMBC can exist in a liminal space in which anti-donation rhetoric argues that solo women have an obligation not to conceive due to producing disadvantaged children despite research in contemporary family studies evidencing similar outcomes for both donor-conceived people and those raised in traditional families.[13] Now, I turn to examine how solo mothers access fertility treatment. In the UK, SMBC are fortunate to have access to fertility treatment and gamete donation as single patients. Although finding and paying for treatment is not necessarily an easy endeavour, there are less barriers than Natsuko faced in *Breasts and Eggs*. However, while there is greater inclusivity for solo women and same sex couples in fertility clinics, these spaces are designed with heterosexual couples in mind. I suggest that even the spaces which offer SMBC support are not free from bias towards the nuclear family. Even though SMBC find sanctuary in the fertility clinic—a space (almost always) diametrically opposed to anti-donation and anti-assisted reproduction narratives—this sanctuary is not without complication; I suggest that liminality also occurs when SMBC feel welcomed into a space that does not seem designed for them.

In the UK, NHS-funded fertility treatment is common for heterosexual couples (and more recently same-sex couples) while solo mothers have 'had the lowest levels of NHS funding in the UK at 6% for IVF and 2% for DI [donor insemination]' (Human Fertilisation and Embryology Authority 2020). This, I suggest, is because solo women often do not fit common reproduction narratives which concentrate on conception failure through natural conception (sexual intercourse); a failure which is often framed as worthy of financial investment and treatment. Furthermore, despite an evolution in how family is formulated, presented, and articulated in our contemporary, the prioritisation of the heterosexual couple persists not because they account, statistically, for the more socially normative reproductive pathway but because they are construed as the healthier pathway. As Jane Juffer in her cultural study on single motherhood remarks, 'the medical establishment and the legal system still assume heterosexual couples make the best parents' (2006, 5).

As noted in the previous chapter, American anthropologist Sarah Franklin notes that '[b]y replicating "natural" conception, IVF itself became a new technology of sex' (2013, 21). Franklin suggests that the term 'technologies of sex' may 'also be called reproductive technologies' (2013, 48). I, however, suggest there needs to be a separation of terms. The SMBC chooses to conceive beyond the influence of sexuality and sex; and so IUI/IVF is not a technology of sex for the SMBC but a technology of conception. While conception involves the fertilisation of an egg cell by a sperm cell, replicating a biological process that occurs through heterosexual sex, this is substitute for, and not an engagement with, sex. The technologisation is of conception itself and separated from sexual interaction with a partner and separate from how an individual experiences or presents their sexuality. Juffer underscores this point by noting that '[r]eproductive freedom for much of Second Wave Feminism meant the choice to have sex without having a baby. Now we might say that reproductive freedom includes the choice to have a baby without having sex' (Juffer 2006, 207).

When scrutinising how fertility clinics advertise their "technologies of sex", there is a clear lean towards assisting infertile heterosexual couples who have been unlucky as to not conceive through sexual intercourse. This means that other pathways receive little bespoke attention. If I examine my clinic, The Lister Fertility Clinic (a facility through which I had great personal success), bias towards couples is first evident in their language.[14] On the front page of their website, they advertise how their practitioners draw on their 'experience of treating over 2000 couples per year' (HCA 2023e). Frequent mention is given to 'childless couples' which positions the website as couple-facing (HCA 2023a). On their IVF page (2023b) and IUI page (2023c), most language is neutral but reference is still made to couples and partners. Even on their 'Alternative Parenting' page, shared motherhood and surrogacy are covered but solo parenthood does not have its own category. Instead, solo women are mentioned in a paragraph on intra-partner egg donation:

An option for single women and same sex couples. Shared motherhood or intra-partner egg donation use IVF treatment, with one partner donating eggs to her partner, and becomes the 'biological mother.' The other partner carries the baby, and experiences the pregnancy as the 'birth mother.' This enables motherhood to be a shared experience right from conception. (HCA 2023d)

Clearly, intra-partner egg sharing (in which a woman gestates a baby conceived from the egg of her female partner) is not appropriate for single patients; it is not clear why this pathway is offered as an option for single women. Similar omissions and conflation are evident in the advertising materials from other clinics. While Complete Fertility Centre does feature a page for single patients, the downloadable brochure has less representation as all testimonials reflect the experience of couples. Care Fertility's homepage features treatment options to choose from split into those for heterosexual couples, female same-sex couples, and male same-sex couples; single women are not mentioned at all. However, under the 'Donations' option on the homepage single women are awkwardly shoehorned in under IVF With Sperm Donor: 'Sometimes, using your own sperm in your fertility treatment just isn't an option—whether that's because you're having trouble with male fertility, or because you're a single woman or female couple' (Care Fertility 2023). Yes, it is not an option for single women to use their own sperm.[15] Here we can see the odd and convoluted way single women (and lesbian couples) are uncomfortably added to a heterosexually framed narrative.

Broadly speaking, the industry itself is geared towards couples with costs and treatment opportunities designed to reflect the bias of state and economic factors which favour couples (for example, some clinics do not open on a weekend and so the solo patient will lose income to attend a clinic during the working week which a couple might more easily absorb). This is something Jane Juffer notes in *Single Mother: The Emergence of the Domestic Intellectual* when she states that beyond the clinic, insurance policies, laws and funds are 'largely invested in the heterosexually coupled nuclear family' which ultimately raises the question as to whether assisted reproduction is a choice for many solo women even if they are invited (2006, 220). However, the prioritisation of couples is not limited to heterosexual couples. Denise Riley, writing on the stigmatisation of the 'single-parent family', notes a political preference towards couples regarding child rearing:

Alarmed debates in the House of Lords in London have asked whether the implication of the proclaimed advantage for any child in having two parents, not just one, was that two "stable" homosexual parents might be just as good as two heterosexual parents (thus also opening the very strong possibility that two homosexual parents might well be judged superior to one single mother). (2002, fn23)

More recently, in the UK's Women's Health Strategy, a document which was presented to Parliament in Autumn 2022, the Secretary of State for Health and Social Care outlined a ten-year plan to improve the wellbeing and health of females in England. One area of focus in this strategy is fertility. The document confirms that what is colloquially called the 'fertility postcode lottery' is an ongoing problem: 'where you live and whether you are in a heterosexual relationship can affect your level of access to NHS-funded IVF provision (Secretary of State for Health and Social Care 2022). In the language used throughout the document, reference is almost exclusively made to pregnancy options for women in couples. Under '10 year ambitions' the second objective for fertility care is fairer treatment for homosexual couples: 'Over the life of this strategy, we will work with NHS England to address the current geographical variation in access to NHS-funded fertility services across England. Female same-sex couples are able to access NHS-funded fertility services in a more equitable way' (Secretary of State for Health and Social Care 2022). Further, the strategy notes that previous barriers (such as self-funding prior to NHS access) will be lifted for female same-sex couples. Single women and solo motherhood are not mentioned. Female same-sex couples who are not experiencing infertility will be seeking NHS treatment to conceive through IUI or IVF with donor sperm, like a solo woman. Yet, although the solo woman would need the same level of treatment, the strategy does not cover support for solo motherhood. In this respect the Women's Health Strategy is making a social, not medical choice and in doing so prioritises co-parenting partnerships. Furthermore, the lack of SMBC representation in policy, advertisements and funding means that some women are unaware of the independent/private options available to them and the potential to pursue solo motherhood (see Chap. 5).

In early 2024, during a Progress Educational Trust (PET) podcast talk on fertility treatment for single people, Dr Sarah Martins da Silva noted that the NHS is designed to provide 'impartial and non-judgemental' treatment but that in terms of fertility treatment 'access is apparently restricted.' Restrictions are partly due to costs but also because NHS treatment criteria is complex. Martins da Silva explains that 'the reality is if you are single there is no NHS funding' but argues that, cost aside, 'the NHS should be accessible to all'. Furthermore, she questions how and why treatment for single people is different than for couples when much of the treatment is the same: 'Young single people have a really good prognosis for fertility and we shouldn't be excluding them by calling them single and not treating them' (in Norcross 2024).

From private clinic to publicly funded programmes, the prioritisation of couples means a disorientating experience for patients who do not fit that model. Although Helen Allan notes that the fertility clinic can be interpreted as a 'safe place' for infertile women to encounter women with similar/shared experiences (2007), this is not necessarily the case for SMBC who often do not find their pathway adequately reflected in NHS provision, policy, and private care. The solo parent is very much in an "in-between" place where clinics represent a safe and inclusive space by providing treatment but simultaneously not a bespoke space in which the SMBC feels adequately represented. How communication can be encouraged and facilitated between clinics and patient community groups is important. As I will explore in Chap. 5, by looking at memoir, auto writing, autoethnography, and interview we can positively destabilise the hierarchical experience in clinical settings in which consultations are 'top down' and reshape the relationship between the fertility industry and recipient communities, so they are more dialogic. This means rethinking the traditional consultation experience in which doctors advise treatment pathways; I suggest that these pathways need to be informed not just by clinical expertise but by consultation with the very communities these clinics are treating. It is important for clinics to appreciate that some SMBC are not entering the clinical space for infertility problems but because they need access to gametes; however, this does not mean that there are not complex feelings associated with the solo mothering pathway. It can be daunting to enter a clinical space that is not necessarily designed inclusively; the solo patient can experience feelings of loss and bereavement for a pathway they either did not want to choose or one that is positioned as inherently problematic.

LIMINAL EXPERIENCE: AMBIGUOUS LOSS

In this section, I will examine the ambiguous loss that SMBC can experience in relation to fertility treatment. As noted, many solo mothers enter fertility clinics settings not because of biological infertility but because they need access to sperm.[16] Some scholars describe this as "social infertility" which means the inability to become pregnant due to a missing gamete component (example: Lo and Campo-Engelstein, 2018).[17] Already, I have shown how feelings of liminality can occur when SMBC engage with fertility clinics and funding that have been designed with couples in mind (and continue to prioritise this parenting structure). Here, I want look at another type of liminal experience: that is of loss. As with any person who experiences involuntary childlessness, there is a sense of bereavement for many SMBC. There may be feelings of loss associated with starting a family without a partner. Financial impossibilities can also represent loss as some solo women cannot access treatment due to the staggering costs of IUI or IVF and their related packages. In her book *Grief Unseen*, Laura Seftel remarks that '[t]here are different kinds of pregnancy loss, including failed in vitro fertilization, molar pregnancy, ectopic pregnancy, loss in multiple-gestation pregnancy, abortion, miscarriage, stillbirth, and others that don't fall easily into one simple category' (2006, 27). I suggest that we should also think of the loss associated with involuntary childlessness experienced by single women. This section focuses on exploring reproductive loss as an ambiguous thing that does not only involve infertility and pregnancy loss but a whole spectrum of grief that is often overlooked or rarely discussed.

While reproductive loss is often associated with pregnancy loss, there is also loss associated with needing to incorporate reproductive technologies into a conception pathway already framed as unethical by some:

> The loss of one's dreams of having a child in a particular way, or of having a child at all, is perhaps the most invisible in the range of reproductive crises, and yet it can be the most consuming of time and emotional energy. (Seftel 2006, 45)

Yet, infertility—most of the time at least—is invisible and unknown; a problem that manifests only when fertility is tested by trying to conceive. Solo people having increasingly popular fertility MOTs (fertility checkups) may discover dwindling fertility, a limited ovarian reserve, and other issues related to conception such as thyroid problems.[18] Data can mark an obscure loss that is hidden within the genetic fibre of a person's being and even foreshadow a loss for those who discover that trying to conceive may be difficult or that pregnancy might be hard to sustain. For couples or co-parenting families struggling with infertility, the plethora of invasive tests trying to locate the root of a problem and then negotiate a plan to overcome reproductive hurdles may involve feelings of loss: loss of control, the loss of the intimacy in the process through the widening of the conception team, and the loss associated with failed conception attempts. Connected to loss is perhaps also a sense of failure—not only of the body failing to produce success but the failure of tests, the failure to ovulate, the failure of the cervix and so on. For the solo parent, there may also be a loss associated with embarking on a less traditional journey without the presence of a partner or co-parent. Unfortunately, if the solo mother is not considered to be part of fertility discourse, loss can also be felt through lack of bespoke care and support.

Yet, there is considerable social and cultural pressure on women to conceive and become mothers because 'Childbearing is the most consistent of human events' and is often presented as a route to completion (Raphael-Leff 2000, 8). In an article in *Time* magazine a surgeon details her experiences with egg freezing in her late 30s and her panic that she might not be able to have children. She said she thought during the harvesting process, 'What is the point of my existence if I cannot perform this basic human function: reproduction?' (Salles 2019). Tracey Loughran and Gayle Davis draw attention to what we might call "motifs of motherhood" through the marketing and saturation of products designed to assist women in conceiving. Every day, from television advertisements to supermarket aisles, women are offered fertility apps, ovulation trackers, pregnancy tests, and supplements which contribute to 'shopping baskets of hope and despair' (Loughran and Davis 2017, 143). Therefore, processing involuntary childlessness is made that much harder due to the dominance successful conception narratives have in society.

Even if parenthood is achieved, there can still be a sense of loss. In M. L. Steenberg et al.'s (2021) pilot study of solo women undergoing medically assisted reproduction in Demark, they note that in their sample 'The women would have preferred to have a child in a relationship with a partner and the shattered dream about the nuclear family has caused a wide range of experiences and emotions.' In a Swedish study on solo parenthood the solo mother is often depicted as 'a woman who unwillingly stands without a co-parent' (Psouni et al. 2022, 1). Many women who pursue SMBC as a 'Plan B' (a route chosen when the first choice of family planning did not work out) have been described as begrudgingly proceeding with fertility assistance based on age concerns (Koert et al. 2022). The pressure of the "biological clock" and fearing developing fertility issues with the passing of time can provoke a woman to seek solo motherhood feeling a certain amount of duress.

Combined, these issues may mean that a solo parent could mourn the loss of their desired family arrangement. This can extend to mourning over a desired number of children. As Emily Koert et al. note, 'Regardless of relationship status, women described feeling grief and regret that they were unable to achieve their desired family size' (2022, 962). Often finances and advancing age can necessitate one child as opposed to fulfilling a desire for more children. Koert et al. call the longing for a specific family formation a 'family clock' (2022, 962). The struggles and trauma of fertility treatment, therefore, are not dispelled with viable pregnancy and live birth but, instead, remain part of the narrative of reproduction for that individual. As Helen Allan (2007) highlights, women who are infertile remain connected to that narrative even if infertility was temporarily "cured" by the clinic to beget their child. To undergo fertility treatment can be an ambiguous experience; for those who have infertility the conception and birthing of a child will not change that reality but can mask it. In a study on the experiences of infertile women in clinics, Allan found that clinics exist in a liminal space in which their function is to 'cure infertility' and secure a viable pregnancy for their patient/s but, because success rates are not 100%, a liminality exists in which practice and reality can be at odds. Allan observes that clinics provide a space of 'tolerance' for women embarking on fertility treatment outside of traditional pathways and can offer a sympathetic environment for women who may feel 'invisible.' However, Allan notes that for women who do not conceive, then the liminal experience felt through infertility is reinforced as the clinic is, obviously, designed to 'transition' infertile women into fertile patients who can and will conceive and birth a child. This strange coexistence of viable pregnancy and infertility can be disorientating. Likewise, fertile solo mothers who engage in treatment traditionally reserved to remedy infertility may feel disorientated.

With the SMBC pathway, the liminal experience of the clinical space as outlined by Allan can be further extended to think about the other ways in which the solo mother may experience feeling disoriented. The SMBC may feel lost in an ambiguous "no space" in which they are judged as a single mother stigmatised by historical notions of disadvantaged family outcomes but celebrated as a product of contemporary feminist opportunity for reproductive independence. Furthermore, dominant narratives offered by anti-donation groups who argue that donor conception creates 'disadvantaged' children wars with sociological research that suggests donor-conceived offspring are not worse off than "naturally" conceived people. Although the law has changed to allow treatment for SMBC in the UK without assessing the need for a partner of the opposite sex, many clinics (although offering inclusive treatment) seem to be talking to heterosexual couples almost exclusively. Feelings of marginality can be further experienced when SMBC are welcomed into clinical spaces but patient-facing resources are not tailored for their specific treatment pathway. Even the language associated with SMBC (Solo Mothers by *Choice*) can create feelings of liminality as many women who opt for gamete donation as a Plan B pathway feel that this was a matter of no choice. As I will explore further in Chap. 5, many SMBC mourn the loss of the "fairy-tale" happy ending in which a family is typically a nuclear one. The mourning of not finding "Prince Charming" is partly rooted in the longing for a romantic partnership but also partly rooted in the societal and cultural narratives that, as I have shown in this chapter, attempt to position partnered parents as a preferable family formation.

Conclusion

Although the cyborg can be viewed as a positive, liberational, and powerful opening up of formerly restrictive understandings of identity and family that has allowed the SMBC to thrive as both technologically assisted and contributing to new social realities of parenting, there are ways in which SMBC can "fall into" problematic gulfs. The SMBC can feel confused, displaced, overlooked, or stigmatised due to the inconsistent way the solo parent is represented in anti-donation discourse and in clinical settings. In summation, reproduction is seen morally as ideally the domain of the heterosexual couple; the couple is also prioritised within infertility clinics designed to treat male/female infertility issues, and—as a result of these two factors—there can be a sense of liminality and ambiguous loss associated with trying to conceive solo. I suggest that these gulfs manifest because of the continued prioritisation of the couple and specifically the male/female nuclear family formation.

Even the celebrated novel *Breasts and Eggs* experiences pressure from the prioritisation of the nuclear family. In my reflection at the start of this chapter, I noted how I first read the novel during maternity leave and was struck by how carefully the author negotiated the SMBC pathway (a point I stand by). However, when I taught the text last year (2023) I discovered something new. I taught the novel for a class on Medical Humanities and was prepared for questions about selfishness and disadvantage. But, when discussing the radical actions of Natsuko, who chose solo motherhood when living in a country that forbade treatment for single women, a student said something that I did not expect and that made me revaluate everything: 'Natsuko wasn't radical, though' she said, 'Natsuko was forced back into nuclear normalcy.'

We all returned to the source material and re-read the final couple of pages. I had always been so focused on the donor conception debate in the book and conversations around selfishness, I had not given much attention to the birth of Natsuko's child. Natsuko was only able to pursue solo motherhood because her known donor attended the clinic with her in a guise of being her romantic partner. 'So, in a way,' the student reasoned, 'she wasn't free at all.' I re-read the book's conclusion on the way home from work—the student was right. There it was on page 422: 'Toward the end of February 2018, we visited an infertility specialist, under the pretence of being in a common law marriage' (Kawakami 2020, 422). How free was Natsuko when she had to become part of the very system she had been pushing against?

In the next chapter, I look at how solo mothers are represented in fiction (film, television, novels and short stories). I will return to Natsuko then as I think about how literature addresses the "blasphemy" of choosing solo motherhood by either casting solo mothers as reckless, selfish, and negligent (therefore obligated not to conceive) or enfolding them back into heterosexual nuclear frameworks in an effort to legitimise the donor-conceived child. We will see how the anti-donation rhetoric and the prioritisation of heterosexual couples covered in this chapter bleed into contemporary popular culture works. Although Natsuko does defy patriarchal state pressures and pursues solo motherhood despite Japanese law forbidding it, we are also reminded that she continues to inhabit a very stigmatised space. As Natsuko's friend Rie notes: 'There's nothing out there for a good-for-nothing single mother' (Kawakami 2020, 252).

NOTES

1. The conference was *Future Directions in Surrogacy Law!* (30 November, 2022) at the Institute of Advanced Legal Studies, London. Golombok's keynote was entitled, "Children Born Through Surrogacy: A Longitudinal Study of Psychological Wellbeing and Relationships with Parents from Age1-Age21".

2. I first wrote about David J. Velleman in "Fatherlessness, sperm donors and 'so what?' parentage: arguing against the immorality of donor conception through 'world literature'", *British Medical Journal: Medical Humanities*, 25 April 2022. https://doi.org/10.1136/medhum-2021-012328 (part of the ISSF/Wellcome Cyborg Conception funded project).

3. However, while the recommendations are that donors should be regulated and non-anonymous, there are cases in the US and with informal donation in the UK where these recommendations are not always observed.

4. On the point of privilege, when Mary Harrington talks about the privileged benefitting from the cyborg, she overlooks her own privilege; in writing about being a "stay at home mother" while her partner financially provides for the family, she neglects to consider the women who must seek alternate options (2023a, 24). While Harrington finds a solution in a strategic marriage to a reliable man, many women do not want or cannot obtain that directed "ideal".

5. XY is reference to the fact that biological boys/men have XY sex chromosomes.

6. Although, I would argue that SMBC is not a compromise at all; it is an alternate model of family configuration.

7. To elaborate, the UK sperm donor donates without financial reward (only the option of recuperation of costs up to £35) and therefore is often framed as an altruistic donor. While the reasons for donation are complex and varied, what is assured is that the donor is not financially benefiting from donation. The recipient of UK donor gametes understands this and therefore interprets the donation as altruistic and not monetised. When money is exchanged between the recipient and the gamete bank/clinic, this is for the service associated with the donation (costs for the bank/clinic include testing, design of profile, preparing and storage of gametes, procedures etc.). It is therefore possible for the act of donation to be seen as separate from the paid process of procedure.

8. Countries in which donor conception is permitted should endeavour to phase out completely anonymous donations and to limit the number of families assisted by each donor.

9. Christine Overall dedicates a chapter of *Why Have Children?* to exploring this issue, concluding that limiting procreation is important, especially in the era of 'procreative carelessness' as represented by the pervasiveness of

shows like *I Didn't Know I Was Pregnant* and shows featuring excessively large families including *Jon and Kate Plus Eight*, *Kate Plus Eight*, *Table for Twelve*, and *Nineteen Kids and Counting* (2012, 176).

10. Many SMBC do choose to adopt.

11. See interviews with Nicola and Sam in Chap. 5.

12. Mary Harrington (Feminism Against Progress) identifies that technology can cause divides (the haves and the have nots, for example) (2023b). This is an important point because gamete donation happens within a complicated industry. While I am focusing on the regulated UK market in which donors cannot sell their gametes, this is still a market in which some women can afford to participate and others cannot. I see the limitations and problems and do not shy away from them: donations should be non-anonymous, donations should have a global limit, and all women—regardless of relationship status—should have access to equal funding.

13. If raised with awareness of their donor conception origins.

14. Of course, the biggest treatment group will be couples and so it is understandable that clinics will market towards couples. However, as solo women do account for one of the largest groups purchasing and using donor sperm it is problematic not to reflect all patient groups adequately on the website.

15. It is possible for clinic issued materials and resources to be more inclusive. Clinics like CREATE Fertility manage to feel more inclusive by referring to treatment options broadly for women often without assuming circumstance (for example, assuming relationship status or sexuality). Likewise, Manchester Fertility speaks broadly to 'patient groups' and one of their key testimonials is from SMBC life coach Melanie Johnson. The website for the Centre for Reproductive and Genetic Health even allows patients to specify not only if they are a single patient but to tailor their experience on the website by selecting whether they are a single man, woman, or transgender person.

16. This is in most cases; however, many solo mothers may need egg donation as well and some may opt for embryo donation. Some solo mothers are aware of pre-existing fertility problems or may become aware of unknown issues when trying to conceive.

17. I prefer the term involuntary childlessness because social infertility suggests a failure to find a partner (the implication with this term is that the woman has failed as a social being to connect romantically). While it may well be the case that some SMBC would have preferred to start a family with a partner, the term social infertility is unnecessarily negative. Instead, whether Plan A or Plan B, SMBC pursue gamete donation because they are childless and not by choice; they actively choose to rectify this by becoming solo parents through sperm donation, double donation, or embryo adoption.

18. Even when an infertility diagnosis is not an issue, age related pressures may present IVF as a more viable pathway than the less invasive and cheaper IUI (insemination) route. The decision to choose IVF knowing it can have hormonal, physical and psychological ramifications as well as contributing to pregnancy and birth complications can be overwhelming. Not to mention that, for many single patients, IVF involves significant time sacrifice which might not be compatible with employment.

References

Allan, H. 2007. Experiences of Infertility: Liminality and the Role of the Fertility Clinic. *Nursing Inquiry* 14(2): 132–139. https://doi.org/10.1111/j.1440-1800.2007.00362.x. Accessed July 16, 2023.

Almond, B. 2006. *The Fragmenting Family.* Oxford: Clarendon.

Austin, M.W. 2007. *Conceptions of Parenthood: Ethics and the Family.* London: Routledge.

Browning, D.S. 2003. *Marriage and Modernization: How Globalization Threatens Marriage and What to Do about It.* Grand Rapids: Eerdmans.

———. 2007. *Equality and the Family: A Fundamental, Practical Theology of Children, Mothers, and Fathers in Modern Societies.* Cambridge: Eerdmans.

Cahn, N.R. 2009. *Test Tube Families. Why the Fertility Market Needs Legal Regulation.* New York: New York University Press.

———. 2013. *The New Kinship: Constructing Donor-Conceived Families.* London: New York University Press.

Callahan, S. 1998. The Ethical Challenge of the New Reproductive Technology. In *Health Care Ethics: Critical Issues for the 21st Century*, ed. J.F. Monagle and D.C. Thomasma. Gaithersburg: Aspen Publishers.

———. 2013. A Life of Mothering. *AMA Journal of Ethics.* https://journalofethics.ama-assn.org/article/life-mothering/2013-09. Accessed January 5, 2021.

Care Fertility. 2023. Donation with Care. https://www.carefertility.com/donation/. Accessed February 28, 2024.

Dahl, R. 1979. *My Uncle Oswald.* London: Penguin.

Davis-Floyd, R., and J. Dumit, eds. 1998. *Cyborg Babies: From Techno-Sex to Techno-Tots.* London: Routledge.

Di Nucci, E. 2016. IVF, Same-Sex Couples and the Value of Biological Ties. *Journal of Medical Ethics* 42(12): 784–787. https://www.jstor.org/stable/44606013. Accessed February 19, 2021.

Evans, E., and C. Grant, eds. 2008. *Mama, PhD: Women Write About Motherhood and Academic Life.* NJ: Rutgers University Press.

Franklin, S. 2013. *Biological Relatives. IVF, Stem Cells, and the Future of Kinship.* London: Duke University Press.

Furse, A. 2001. *Your Essential Infertility Companion: A User's Guide to Tests, Technology and Therapies.* London: Thorsons.

Golombok, S. 2015a. *Modern Families: Parents and Children in New Family Forms.* Cambridge: Cambridge University Press.

———. 2015b. Children Do Just as Well in 'New Family Structures' as in the Traditional Family. *Children and Family blog.* https://childandfamilyblog. com/new-family-structures/#:~:text=The%20research%20simply%20 shows%20that%20they%20are%20just,raised.%20That%20includes%20 society%E2%80%99s%20attitudes%20towards%20the%20family.   Accessed March 4, 2023.

Golombok, S., E. Ilioi, L. Blake, G. Roman, and V. Jadva. 2017. A Longitudinal Study of Families Formed Through Reproductive Donation: Parent-Adolescent Relationships and Adolescent Adjustment at Age 14. *Developmental Psychology* 53(10): 1966–1977. https://psycnet.apa.org/fulltext/2017-32863-001.pdf. Accessed January 12, 2021.

Graham, S. 2018. Being a 'Good' Parent: Single Women Reflecting Upon 'Selfishness' and 'Risk' When Pursuing Motherhood Through Sperm Donation. *Anthropology & Medicine* 25: 249–264.

Harrington, M. 2023a. *Feminism Against Progress.* Croydon: Forum.

———. 2023b. The Contraceptive Tetrad. *Reactionary Feminist,* November 18. https://reactionaryfeminist.substack.com/p/the-contraceptive-tetrad. Accessed February 16, 2024.

HCA (HCA Healthcare UK). 2023a. Being an Egg Donor. https://www.hca-healthcare.co.uk/our-services/treatments/being-an-egg-donor.   Accessed November 15, 2023.

———. 2023b. In Vitro Fertilisation (IVF). https://www.hcahealthcare.co.uk/our-services/treatments/in-vitro-fertilisation-ivf. Accessed November 15, 2023.

———. 2023c. Intrauterine Insemination (IUI). https://www.hcahealthcare. co.uk/our-services/treatments/intrauterine-insemination-iui.   Accessed November 15, 2023.

———. 2023d. Shared Motherhood. https://www.hcahealthcare.co.uk/our-services/treatments/alternative-parenting/shared-motherhood.   Accessed November 15, 2023.

———. 2023e. Welcome to the Lister Fertility Clinic. https://www.hcahealth-care.co.uk/facilities/the-lister-hospital/units-and-teams/lister-fertility-clinic. Accessed November 15, 2023.

Human Fertilisation and Embryology Authority. 1990. Human Fertilisation and Embryology Authority Act 1990. https://www.legislation.gov.uk/ ukpga/1990/37/pdfs/ukpga_19900037_en.pdf. Accessed January 12, 2021.

———. 2020. Family Formations in Fertility Treatment 2018. https://www.hfea. gov.uk/about-us/publications/research-and-data/family-formations-in-fertility-treatment-2018. Accessed March 4, 2021.

Johnson, M. 2020. Going Solo with Genevieve Roberts. *The Stork and I* Podcast. July 8.

Juffer, J. 2006. *Single Mother: The Emergence of the Domestic Individual*. London: New York University Press.

Kawakami, M. 2020. *Breasts and Eggs. Translated by Sam Bett and David Boyd*. New York: Picador.

Koert, E., R. Sylvest, I. Vittrup, H.W. Hvidman, K.B. Peterson, J. Boivin, A.N. Anderson, and L. Schmidt. 2022. The Importance of the 'Family Clock': Women's Lived Experience of Fertility Decision-making 6 Years after Attending the Fertility Assessment and Counselling Clinic. *Human Fertility* 25 (5): 954–966.

Layne, L.L. 2013. 'Creepy,' 'Freaky,' and 'Strange': How the 'Uncanny' Can Illuminate the Experience of Single Mothers by Choice and Lesbian Couples Who Buy 'Dad'. *Journal of Consumer Culture* 13 (2): 140–159.

———. 2015. I Have a Fear of Really Screwing It Up: The Fears, Doubts, Anxieties, and Judgments of One American Single Mother by Choice. *Journal of Family Issues* 36: 1154–1170.

Lewis, B.C. 2012. *Papa's Baby: Paternity and Artificial Insemination*. London: New York University Press.

Lo, W., and L. Campo-Engelstein. 2018. Expanding the Clinical Definition of Infertility to Include Socially Infertile Individuals and Couples. In *Reproductive Ethics II*, ed. L. Campo-Engelstein and P. Burcher. Cham: Springer. https://doi.org/10.1007/978-3-319-89429-4_6. Accessed November 12, 2022.

Loughran, T., and G. Davis. 2017. Introduction: The Body Politic and the Infertile Body. In *The Palgrave Handbook of Infertility in History: Approaches, Contexts and Perspectives*, ed. Gayle Davis and Tracey Loughran, 143–149. Palgrave Macmillan.

Mack, K. 2020. I Am Murphy Brown: Race and Class in Rhetorics of Single Mothers by Choice. *Rhetoric Review* 39 (3): 287–302.

Monosson, E. 2008. *Motherhood, The Elephant in the Laboratory*. London: ILR Press.

Morrissette, M. 2008. *Choosing Single Motherhood: The Thinking Woman's Guide*. New York: Houghton Mifflin Company.

Norcross, S. 2024. PET Podcast: Fertility Treatment for Single People—Who Should Pay? *PET*, January 29. https://www.progress.org.uk/pet-podcast-fertility-treatment-for-single-people-who-should-pay/. Accessed February 16, 2024.

Overall, C. 2012. *Why Have Children?: The Ethical Debate*. London: MIT Press.

Parke, R.D. 2013. *Future Families: Diverse Forms, Rich Possibilities*. Oxford: John Wiley & Sons.

Psouni, E., J. Berg, and H. Persson. 2022. 'Solo Mothers' By Choice Experiences During Pregnancy and Early Parenthood: Thoughts and Feelings Related To Maternal Health-services. *Sexual and Reproductive Healthcare Elsevier*. 33: 1–6.

Raphael-Leff, J., ed. 2000. *Spilt Milk: Perinatal Loss and Breakdown*. London: Taylor & Francis.

Ravn, T. 2021. *Lived Realities of Solo Motherhood, Donor Conception and Medically Assisted Reproduction*. Emerald Studies in Reproduction, Culture and Society.

Renvoize, J. 2023. *Going Solo: Single Mothers by Choice*. London: Routledge.

Riley, D. 2002. The Right to be Lonely. *Differences: A Journal of Feminist Cultural Studies* 13 (1): 1–13.

Roth, A. 2016. What Does Queer Family Equality Have To Do With Reproductive Ethics? *International Journal of Feminist Approaches to Bioethics*, 9(1): 27–67. https://www.jstor.org/stable/10.2307/90011857. Accessed March 2, 2021.

Salles, A. 2019. I Spent My Fertile Years Training to Be a Surgeon. Now, It Might Be Too Late for Me to Have a Baby. *Time*, January 3. https://time.com/5484506/fertility-egg-freezing/. Accessed August 12, 2020.

Schmidt, M., and L.J. Moore. 1998. Constructing a 'Good Catch,' Picking a Winner. In *Cyborg Babies: From Techno-Sex to Techno-Tots*, ed. R. Davis-Floyd and J. Dumit, 21–39. London: Routledge.

Schneider, D.M. 1968. *American Kinship: A Cultural Account*. London: University of Chicago Press.

Secretary of State for Health and Social Care. 2022. Women's Health Strategy. August 30, 2022, CP 736. https://www.gov.uk/government/publications/womens-health-strategy-for-england/womens-health-strategy-for-england. Accessed December 2, 2023.

Seftel, L. 2006. *Grief Unseen: Healing Pregnancy Loss Through the Arts*. London: Jessica Kingsley.

Solomon, J., and C. George. 2006. Intergenerational Transmission of Dysregulated Maternal Caregiving: Mothers Describe Their Upbringing and Childrearing. In *Parenting Representations: Theory, Research, and Clinical Implications*, ed. Ofra Mayseless, 265–295. Cambridge: Cambridge University Press.

Somerville, M. 2011. Donor Conception and Children's Rights: 'First, Do No Harm'. *Canadian Medical Association Journal* 183(2). https://doi.org/10.1503/cmaj.101388. Accessed February 16, 2021.

Steenberg, M.L., R. Sylvest, E. Koert, and L. Schmidt. 2021. P-472 Single Mothers by Choice—Experiences of Single Women Seeking Treatment at a Public Fertility Clinic in Denmark: A Pilot Study. *Human Reproduction* 36 (Suppl. 1). https://doi.org/10.1093/humrep/deab130.471.

The Ethics Committee of the American Society for Reproductive Medicine. 2013. *Access to Fertility Treatment by Gays, Lesbians, and Unmarried Persons: A Committee Opinion* 100 (6). https://www.asrm.org/globalassets/asrm/asrm-content/news-and-publications/ethics-committee-opinions/access_to_fertility_treatment_by_gays_lesbians_and_unmarried_persons-pdfmembers.pdf. Accessed March 4, 2021.

Vandenberg-Daves, J. 2014. *Modern Motherhood: An American History*. New Brunswick: Rutgers University Press.

Velleman, J.D. 2015a. Family History. In *Beyond Price: Essays on Birth and Death*, 1st ed., 61–78. Cambridge: Open Book Publishers. http.//www.jstor.org/stable/j.ctt17w8gwg.7. Accessed March 4, 2023.

———. 2015b. Introduction. In *Beyond Price: Essays on Life and Death*. Cambridge: Open Book Publishers, 1–3. https://www-jstor-org.ezproxy.lib.bbk.ac.uk/stable/pdf/j.ctt17w8gwg.3.pdf?refreqid=fastly-default%3A8d493c c0bb1553950804591d73a7c5e8&ab_segments=&origin=&initiator=&accep tTC=1. Accessed March 4, 2023.

———. 2015c. Persons in Prospect. In *Beyond Price: Essays on Life and Death*. Cambridge: Open Book Publishers, 79–139. https://www-jstor-org.ezproxy.lib.bbk.ac.uk/stable/pdf/j.ctt17w8gwg.8.pdf?refreqid=fastly-default%3Afca7 7906b6fcc792f307b16e380d21ad&ab_segments=&origin=&initiator=&acce ptTC=1. Accessed March 4, 2023.

CHAPTER 4

Reckless Radicals: The Solo Mother in Fiction and Popular Culture

Abstract In this chapter, I explore how the Solo Mother by Choice (SMBC) is presented in mainstream film, television, and literature which have traditionally been preoccupied with dichotomies, notably the nuclear family utopia pitted against single-parent dystopia. Why does the "happy ever after" in fiction featuring solo mothers necessitate romance? In what ways is romance used as a plot device to "correct" the problem of solo parenting?

Keywords Assisted reproduction • Cyborg • Family • Fairy tale • Fatherlessness • Fertility • Fiction • Film • Gamete donation • Goddess • Literature • Nuclear family • Selfishness • Single mother • Solo mother • Stereotype • Stigma • Television

REFLECTION

> Donor insemination has not been normalised in the media the way other forms of single mothering have been, indicating that the 'public' still views assisted technology as not quite natural. (Juffer 2006, 228)

There was a very specific moment in which I realised I wanted to research conception storytelling and that was when I was reading Beatrix Potter's *The Tale of Jemima Puddle-Duck* (1908) to my toddler children. I vaguely knew the Potter characters: Mr. Jeremy Fisher, Mrs. Tiggy-winkle, Flopsy,

G. Halden, *Cyborg Conception*,
https://doi.org/10.1007/978-3-031-59386-4_4

Mopsy, and Cotton-tail, etc. I only knew them as their animals: the frog, the hedgehog, and the rabbits. Jemima I simply knew as the duck who encountered a fox. However, I was surprised to read that Jemima, penned and illustrated in 1908, is a solo mother by choice.

The story goes that Jemima left her farm to embark on motherhood solo: 'I wish to hatch my own eggs; I will hatch them all by myself' (Potter [1908] 2013, 7). I smiled as I read this line to my twins, finding it endearing but amusing to identify with a fictitious duck. On her journey to find a safe place to deliver and hatch her eggs, Jemima comes across a 'foxy gentleman'. With a low-pitched voice, I attempted a tone that would sound both charismatic but menacing; I rasped, 'Madam, have you lost your way?' (Potter [1908] 2013, 12). My children were too young to appreciate the danger that Jemima was in, but I was all too aware that her choice to follow the fox home would be a costly mistake. My eyes skimmed ahead to see that, sure enough, the seductive fox would attempt to devour both the duck and her offspring.

While I playfully manipulated my voice for the high-pitched Jemima and the sultry fox, my mind was busily decoding the metaphors. Or rather, identifying themes I was reading into the story as a SMBC via sperm donation. While to my children the fox was merely a fox, to me I read him as a predatory masculine force who lures Jemima in with the promise to help her birth ducklings. He reminded me of unscrupulous unregulated online donors with their posts on Facebook offering "natural insemination" in a hotel and promises of a guaranteed pregnancy due to their high success rate of siring offspring in the hundreds. To me the parallels were clear: a fox described as having virility (he is a 'bushy long-tailed gentleman') and described as offering a paternal role (of sorts): 'He said he loved eggs and ducklings; he should be proud to see a fine nestful in his woodshed' (Potter [1908] 2013, 18).

Perhaps predictably, Jemima does lose her eggs (although to a pack of puppies, which was a surprise) and this miscarriage is a sombre read in a book aimed at children. By the end of the tale, Jemima has successfully hatched her chicks. While this is a happy moment, and I pointed out the brood to my twins as evidence of success, Potter identified one last inadequacy for poor Jemima: she hatched only four eggs. The average clutch, I'm told, is eight to fourteen. This Jemima blames on herself: 'Jemima Puddle-duck said that it was because of her nerves; but she had always been a bad sitter' (Potter [1908] 2013, 29). Poor Jemima, I empathised: so many women blame themselves for not producing enough eggs during IVF rounds.

When my boys fell asleep, I flicked through the book again, noticing this time that each page is decorated at the border with four ducklings, representative of the four chicks Jemima was destined to hatch. Those chicks haunt Jemima on every page. At the top of the page they represent her dreams, and at the bottom of the page they represent an anchor—something from which she could not move on. The duckling in each corner of the page contains the narrative within a frame like a fence which entraps Jemima's suffering, loss, and grief. The successful hatching at the end brings the four ducklings from peripheral spectre to present success. A happy moment.

In noticing this detail, I started to think about how parents today narrativise and frame their reproduction pathways. My friend Stephanie, who had IVF to conceive her twins with her husband, kept a photo journal of her journey from medication to blastocyst to scan to birth. When my babies spent four weeks in the neonatal intensive care unit, I did the same: I kept a photo journal of their progression from incubator to cot to discharge. I found, as did Stephanie, that storytelling and images became a therapeutic way of processing uncertainty and trauma linked to reproduction and birth.

With reproductive imaging, Stephanie was able to form a connection with the blastocysts that would become her children. The heart she drew on her ultrasound in pink digital marker became, months later, reimagined in a photoshoot of her twins framed by the needles and medications that underpinned her IVF; this imaging does not tell a story of invasive and intrusive technology but of collaboration. The ability to become familiar with the blastocyst and embryo can help create intimacy between patient and process; the mediation of technology becomes less intrusive when an image records and projects ownership of a developing embryo that is associated with beginnings and family. For Stephanie's children, this photo diary will also demystify their origin story.

Storytelling is an important method through which to therapeutically navigate conception crises, but it is also an important method through which to explore non-traditional reproduction routes. The need to demystify and normalise families created through assisted reproduction has resulted in the publication of many independent books created by and for families formed through sperm/egg/embryo donation. One of the first books I bought for my children was *Our Story: How We Became a Family* (Barnsley and Clarkson 2018), published by the Donor Conception Network. This book narrates the story of a solo mother to twins through sperm donation. Now our bookshelf is crammed with books about different families; popular bedtime choices include *The Great Big Book of Families* (Hoffman and Asquith 2010) and *The Family Book* (Parr 2010), both of which gently educate children about diverse family structures including solo parent families.

What is it that I read? You would think, following the increase in treatment for solo women since the 1980s, that solo motherhood by choice would be well represented in contemporary fiction. It isn't—well, not positively anyway. So, I find myself still thinking about Jemima; the SMBC who is described as 'quite desperate' and 'determined to make a nest right away' (Potter [1908] 2013, 8). The duality of the solo mother as desperate/determined, I would come to discover, is very common in adult fiction featuring SMBC. Remember this line, for it shall define this chapter: 'Jemima Puddle-duck was a simpleton' (Potter [1908] 2013, 20). And yes, Mr Fox, it seems that *Madam* has lost her way...

Introduction: What Is Cyborg Fiction?

In this chapter, I turn to look at how the Solo Mother by Choice (SMBC) is represented in mainstream fiction. As I have aligned the SMBC with cyborg conception, it is worth first exploring how the stereotypical cyborg is typically framed in literature before I explain how I am intending to use fiction to explore SMBC characters. Science fiction is the genre most associated with the cyborg. The subgenre of cyberpunk—which became a literary movement in the 1980s around the same time of Donna Haraway's cyborg, Jean Shinoda Bolen's Goddess, and Jane Mattes' solo mother organisation—is perhaps most intimately connected to the trope of the cyborg. Cyberpunk as a term was coined in 1983 in Bruce Bethke's story of the same name. Bethke's story features a protagonist hacker who is cyborg through both their fusion with technology and their environmental conditioning by technology. The subgenre itself is famously known for its dystopian treatment of technology, speculative tales of mechanised societies, the decay of humanity, the destruction of the planet, and the genesis of hybrid beings. Cyberpunk is saturated by "melded" cyborgs such as the weaponised Molly Millions from William Gibson's *Neuromancer* (1984) who prostituted her body in exchange for cybernetic upgrades. In a nutshell, we might associate the 80s cyberpunk movement with ideas of fearsome technologies, the undermining of the sanctity of the human condition, and an apocalyptic future. The victim in cyberpunk is the human who has become oppressed, hybridised, and rendered redundant. New life rises in the form of hybrid entities, artificial intelligences, and nanotechnology. Even theoretical writing on the cyborg tends to reflect on the cyborg in science fiction. In *Cyborg Babies*, Robbie Davis-Floyd and Joseph Dumit note the dominance of the cyborg in popular culture 'From the Six-Million-Dollar man to the Terminator' (1998, 1). They explain that '[w]e are immersed in cyborgs; they saturate our language, our media, our technology', as well as the ways in which we understand humanness and the boundary between enhancement and endangerment (1998, 1). Likewise, posthumanist thinker N. Katherine Hayles notes that literature on the posthuman can be 'obsessed, in various ways, with the dynamics of evolution and devolution' (1999, 281). Here Hayles is speaking about science fiction texts such as *Blood Music* (1983), *Snow Crash* (1992) and *Terminal Games* (1994).

Popular cultural ideas of the cyborg in texts like *Blood Music* and *The Terminator* (1984) are probably what most people think about when they think of cyborg and cyborg fiction. Yet, I find it more interesting to think about the "everyday" cyborg, like the SMBC who represents both technological assistance and (more radically perhaps) a new type of social reality for what reproduction and family can mean today. In fact, when we look at definitions of what the science fiction genre purports to do, we can see that most writing on the SMBC does something very similar. Science fiction has been described as '*ideologically* challenging' (Shippey 2008, 21), 'literature of change' (Landon 2002, xi), 'an ongoing discussion' (Mendlesohn 2007, 10) and 'What If literature' (Russ 1974, 6). In this chapter, I explore how SMBC in fiction is ideologically challenging, how the fiction examines the changing landscape of family construction, and how it contributes to an ongoing discussion on the nature of reproduction and family. A lot of what is under discussion in this book deals with '*What happens if*' issues: *What happens if* women have children solo? *What happens if* people use gamete donation? *What happens if* we incorporate technological intervention into the human reproduction process?

In literature, film and television featuring the SMBC we can see an obsession with the dynamics of evolution and devolution like Hayles described but without exploring the melding of organic and artificial in the technical and fantastical cyborg. In my understanding, the concern over devolution of the nuclear family in SMBC fiction chimes with Donna Haraway's argument that the cyborg is blasphemous. As I explored in the last chapter, the SMBC is bound up in questions surrounding the "unnaturalness" of solo motherhood through gamete donation. The SMBC can be seen to be blasphemous to the natural order of reproduction—as representing disrespect towards the sacredness of the natural. Arguably, with SMBC the blasphemy is the confrontation of choice that poses a threat to the idealism of the heteronormative two-parent family formation.

The desire to protect nuclear family ideals contributed to the unwillingness of fertility clinics to treat unmarried women in the 1970s and 1980s. Consequently, when women choose to "go solo"—to actively choose to become single parents—the decision is often painted as selfish and narcissistic; this is implied in Amadeo D'Adamo and Elaine Hoffman Baruch's work in which the SMBC is argued to represent 'a fantasy of omnipotence-a wish to function as both sexes, to be everything for the child' (1986, 77). This so-called fantasy of omnipotence is punished when women who seek reproductive control are presented as dangerous and fickle. The struggle for positive representation of the solo mother reflects the struggle that comes with any type of writing on the cyborg. Haraway describes 'Cyborg politics' as the 'struggle for language and the struggle against perfect communication' (1991, 176). The struggle of the SMBC to communicate the reality of their conception pathway is further problematised by stigmatising language surrounding both assisted reproduction and single parenthood (both positioned in many literary works as somehow inferior to natural conception by heterosexual couples).

As I have shown in previous chapters, the single mother is often unhelpfully polarised as cyborg or goddess. These archetypes, as Haraway noted, are often 'bound in a spiral dance' (1991, 181). This polarisation reflects how the media represents single mothers as either 'successful career women or young welfare check dependent mothers' (Parke 2013, 233). Writing in the 1980s, in their work on the treatment of the single mother in modern society, Peggy Quinn and Katherine R. Allen note that one solution to the problematic single mother (regardless of circumstance) was marriage, which was viewed as the way to secure a "normal" family (1989, 394). As this chapter will illustrate, the blasphemy of solo parenting (disrespect of the "sacredness" of heterosexual reproduction) is often neutralised through romance and the attainment of the "normal" family. By offering salvation in an eventual heterosexual coupling through which the SMBC is no longer a solo mother, the SMBC is moved away from the liberational cyborg and back into the Demeter goddess archetype. Here, the ideal woman and mother is framed through her connection to a husband and father. While there is increasing inclusivity offered in many twenty-first-century children's books, literature aimed at young adults and adults often presents solo motherhood as dysfunctional, with many solo mothers described as selfish in their determination to conceive and reckless in their desperation for a baby. In this chapter, I will show how SMBC who do not experience the corrective embrace of heteronormative co-parenting in fiction are villainised.

THE "INADEQUATE" SOLO MOTHER IN YOUNG-ADULT LITERATURE

I want to start by examining how the solo mother is presented as an inadequate parent in many young-adult literature (YA) texts featuring gamete donation as a theme. In a lot of YA literature on donor conception, the protagonist, often aged between thirteen and eighteen years old, is a donor-conceived person who grapples either with the fact that they are donor-conceived or grapples with wider issues impacting—and threatening—their family. Although it is essential to consider the experiences of donor-conceived people, many of these narratives are not written by donor-conceived people and instead employ donor conception storylines as a point of narrative interest. In the YA novels to be considered in this chapter, the plots do not necessarily address issues and concerns with donor conception itself but rather with the act of solo mothering. Many of the scenarios presented in these YA texts show the SMBC to be reckless, selfish, negligent, and struggling.

Sociologist Margaret K. Nelson has already done some important work in this area. In the paper 'The Presentation of Donor Conception in Young Adult Fiction', Nelson analysed thirty YA texts that include the theme of donor conception in what she describes as the 'problem novel' or 'coming of age novel' (2019, 37). Nelson found that donor children conceived by SMBC were more likely to be written as endangered despite research indicating that donor-conceived adolescents are 'well-adjusted' (Nelson 2019, 35). However, this endangerment is often not directly related to their conception or their family formation (e.g. in many stories the adolescent's encounter with a stranger places them in danger, see: Jean Gill's *Left Out* 2017, Francis Chalifour's *Call Me Mimi* 2009, Laura Kasischke's *Feathered* 2008).[1] The incidental nature of endangerment, however, does present the donor-conceived child of a SMBC as embedded in a world of trauma, risk, uncertainty, and dysfunction. While Nelson (2019) concludes her survey of donor conception fiction for adolescents with the argument that donor conception is 'normalised' the SMBC is still problematised and sometimes even demonised. For example, in the comedic YA fiction novel *Donuthead* by Sue Stauffacher eleven-year-old Franklin reflects on stereotypical beliefs about single mother families being sites of endangerment:

> My mother is husbandless. This is both devastating and out of my control. I have mentioned to my mother that coming from a single-parent home puts me at a disproportionately high risk for all sorts of life-threatening behaviors, like alcohol and drug abuse, depression and anger management issues, and being abducted by kidnappers on the rare evening she has to work late. (2003, n.p.)

Despite Franklin's mother being a strong and positive parent, her son's statement reveals an underlining concern over disadvantage which has long been associated with single parenting. As Nelson remarks, many YA donor conception stories feature the sentiment that 'single mothers might be better off with a man if not for their own sake, for the sake of their children' (2019, 53). This is because heteronormative gender binaries are upheld: a family should consist of a mother and a father, one to nurture (female) and one to protect (male). The stories in which donor-conceived children face danger could be argued to be partly due to the absence of the father as protector and the inability of the mother to juggle the roles of nurturer, provider, and protector as a solo parent.

Nelson has done a brilliant job in highlighting how donor conception is viewed in YA literature across different family types, but I want to focus specifically here on how SMBC are presented. Nelson notes that in most of the YA literature, 'being donor-conceived does not dictate the plot'— meaning donor-conceived people are written in a complex way and deal with a variety of issues that exist beyond their conception history (2019, 51–52). Yet, I argue that in these texts the solo mother is reduced to a two-dimensional character; she is rarely fleshed out beyond being a single woman or a former solo parent. This means that many SMBC in YA fiction tend to represent negative stereotypes (to various extents). The SMBC is often described by others—usually the donor-conceived person but sometimes an omnipresent narrator—and as a result the reader does not learn about the character's history or motivation for solo mothering first hand. Instead, we learn about the SMBC through the summaries and judgements of other characters.

In many YA texts, the choice of being a SMBC is presented as a flippant and impulsive decision by the children. In Francis Chalifour's *Call Me Mimi* (2009), Mimi's mother is a Plan B SMBC who is described by her child as choosing sperm donation spontaneously: 'When she turned thirty-nine, she divorced the guy, sold the house, coloured her hair blonde, and went to a sperm bank in Toronto' (15). Similar occurs in Emily Franklin's *The Other Half Of Me* (2007) in which the SMBC is described as acting impulsively: 'after a lunch meeting in Santa Monica, my mom visited a doctor's office off of Montana Avenue and picked a donor' (n.p.). In Franklin's text donor conception is presented as an unfortunate premature decision as the mother went on to meet a suitable man during pregnancy who would become the father of her three subsequent children: 'Mom had me back when she was super work-focused and single and thought she'd be alone forever. Of course, she got pregnant (after choosing 142 from the other donors), met my actual dad, and had me. They got married when I was one' (2007, n.p.). There are three implications to how SMBC are characterised here. First, it is suggested that career women must focus either on a family or on their profession; the SMBC is judged as being so 'super work-focused' that they had to pursue a "Plan B" option. Second, when donor conception is mentioned, the mother's choice is surrounded by quote marks to underscore that this "decision" was not one that involved much deliberation (Franklin 2007, n.p.). Third, the fact the SMBC meets a romantic suitor during pregnancy positions SMBC as a hasty decision and one that could have been avoided if she had just been patient.

Although donor conception is presented as a hasty decision in *Call Me Mimi* and *The Other Half Of Me*, both children are born to a loving mother and into a secure and nurturing family environment. When this does not happen, and the child is born into an inadequate environment, the author tends to place the blame for poor mothering on the very fact that the mother is a solo mother. For example, the "reckless" impulse of a SMBC to have a child in Joyce Sweeney's novel *Headlock* is presented as disastrous throughout the novel. Again, we rarely hear from the SMBC directly, but we do learn that her "selfish" drive for motherhood has directly led to the abuse and criminal endangerment of her child. In *Headlock*, the SMBC acts on a whim and then distances herself from mothering after a few years due to dissatisfaction with the responsibility of childcare: 'Mom felt that every woman should experience childbirth, so at forty-three, she picked my dad out of a catalogue and presto—fulfilled! For four years anyway' (2006, n.p.). Reference to a generic "catalogue" but lack of reference to specific donor details recorded on profiles links the decision to the casual act of shopping, commercialisation, and frivolous decision making. The decision to procreate is presented as a selfish act as highlighted by the line 'every woman should experience'; the word 'should' positions the experience as something narcissistic with little reflection on the life that will result. Kyle ends up abandoned by his mother ('My mother's in Connecticut, not raising me') which underscores the message that the SMBC does not consider the life and wellbeing of the resulting child—as does Kyle's realisation that his mother 'found out she didn't want to have a kid' (Sweeney 2006, n.p.). Kyle's mother is portrayed as more interested in romance and the drive to find a love interest overrides any interest in mothering. Kyle's mother is described as unreliable and neglectful with a stream of dysfunctional romantic interests: 'Genaro is the latest in a long line of loser boyfriends, all younger than her, all with dubious entrepreneurial tendencies, which my mom helps fund' (Sweeney 2006, n.p.). Kyle's upbringing was so traumatic that the negative experiences he had with his mother tainted his view on all women: 'Women are vicious tacticians. Don't ever let them fool you' (Sweeney 2006, n.p.). By conceiving solo, his mother is portrayed as a tactician and by abandoning her responsibilities is presented as vicious. Overall, Kyle's mother represents deception: she is deceptive about her motivations to have a child and about her intent on raising a baby solo. The choice to be a solo mother is made, but the pathway becomes too hard and boring to traverse and so she abandons her family.

In several narratives, the SMBC is presented by the author or protagonist as needing to choose solo motherhood because they are undesirable women. Whether being a solo mother is a reckless or dangerous decision aside, this route is sometimes portrayed as the only option for women who are too difficult to secure partnership. In *Feathered*, SMBC Roberta Tompkins is presented as so unlikable that it is suggested she needs to pursue SMBC due to her domineering demeanour: 'She was attractive enough, but so solid and blunt that you could sort of see why it was easier for her to make a baby with a sperm, and a syringe, than with a man, in a bed' (Kasischke 2008, 16). The problem, it is suggested, is that Roberta's personality is too forthright to secure the interest of a decent suitor. In *Left Out*, the first introduction to Ryan's mother is from his critical perspective: 'Ryan was less pleased to find his mother at home' (Gill 2017, n.p.). Ryan's chief complaint is that his educated mother is opinionated and this causes his frustration and embarrassment; Ryan's conception and birth is attributed to his mother's self-righteousness and selfish determination: 'He was the result of her opinions on bringing up children. Worse than that, he was the result of her opinions on the right of a single woman to be a mother' (Gill 2017, n.p).

In her survey of donor conception in YA literature, Nelson (2019) notes there is a lack of sexual educational materials on donor conception for adolescents and so the 'problem novel' fills that gap. This means that adolescents can only really explore donor conception narratives through fiction; because these novels often present outlandish and sensationalised plots adolescents are predominately exposed to parent "problem" narratives rather than a nuanced interpretation of the social, emotional, and psychological contexts of donation. This is extremely problematic as donor-conceived youth receive skewed stories of (as Nelson's research indicates) dangerous single mother trauma narratives. What I believe would be more beneficial for YA audiences are works which explore the complex and nuanced issues and challenges encountered by donor-conceived people as articulated in testimony (see: *We Are Donor Conceived*; Louise McLoughlin's podcast *You Look Like Me* 2020–2023; memoirs like Kiara Schuh's *Chosen Family* 2022; and personal stories from The Donor Conceived Community). It is also important to explore the decisions for choosing solo motherhood through the SMBC themselves, rather than reductively summarise complex choices through the biased lens of another character. Referring to testimony would help to flesh out of these issues (see Chap. 5). Many of the issues presented in these examples of YA literature have less to do with being donor-conceived and more to do with being born, as Franklin states in *Donuthead*, to a 'husbandless' mother. However, what it actually means to be a 'husbandless mother' is never really explored through the mother herself. Instead, she is described and judged at a distance and dismissed as a side-character. In the next section, I will look at how in adult fiction, the "problem" of the solo mother is "corrected" by making her a principal character who is, more often than not, "saved" through finding a partner.

Correcting the "Problem" of the Single Mother in Adult Fiction

In the last chapter, I reflected on my evolved understanding of Mieko Kawakami's novel *Breasts and Eggs* (2020). This novel, which was originally published in 2008 but was not translated into English until 2019, provides an account of how single woman Natsuko wishes to become a solo mother through gamete donation as her first and only choice for family planning. Initially, I interpreted the text as a nuanced account of the pathways to donor conception and a careful articulation regarding the necessitation of non-anonymous sperm donation. However, I soon came to realise that, although Natsuko represents defiance towards the policy in Japan not to provide fertility treatment to single women, she ultimately (and understandably) has to adhere to heteronormative co-parenting ideals to access treatment. Natsuko does this by claiming that her sperm donor is her romantic partner and co-parent. Despite Natsuko's determination to become a Plan A SMBC, she cannot be open about this commitment less she be judged, as her friend Rie warns her, as a 'good-for-nothing single mother' (Kawakami 2020, 252).

In this section, I will look at how SMBC is portrayed across different popular culture texts aimed at adults in both the UK and US. Juffer notes that '[s]ingle mothers on screen now represent the acceptance of some non-traditional households precisely because real single moms can choose—choose to have or raise a baby on their own' (2006, 46). It might be the case that strong single mother figures like Ros from *Fraiser* (1993–2004)[2] receive acceptance, but this is not always true of women in fiction who are penned as irresponsibly choosing solo parenthood pre-conception. I want to consider how mainstream fiction—from television comedy series to crime dramas to romantic fiction—highlight SMBC as problematic and even humorous before "correcting" the "problem" of solo motherhood by enveloping the SMBC back into a nuclear family structure. While Natsuko, arguably, does not have a choice but to present herself as a partner and co-parent to adhere to cultural rules and treatment laws in Japan, in fiction set in post 2000 in UK and US settings, there is no need to enfold the SMBC back into co-parenting models—certainly not unhealthy ones. Why, I wonder, is SMBC "corrective literature" such a trend?

SMBC is popular as a comedic subplot in US television series. In *Friends* (1994–2004), Monica Geller tries different strategies to get over a breakup; one way is to make lots of jam and another way is to become pregnant with a sperm donor. Immediately, the plan is framed as 'stupid' with reference made to Monica sourcing sperm from 'the docks' (Bright 1996). After a day of contemplation, Monica is talked out of her impulsive decision. In *My Crazy Ex-Girlfriend* (2015–2019), "crazy" Rebecca Bunch stalks and attempts to force a woman to act as an egg donor for her solo father friend Darryl, in what is lightly portrayed as harmless, humorous shenanigans. When forcing the woman to donate fails, Rebecca becomes Darryl's egg donor herself—a decision not thoroughly thought out by either party which is highlighted as Darryl frequently laments that Rebecca shows no maternal interest in the child (Rebecca often forgets she even donated). In *Workin' Moms* (2017–2023), Sloane Mitchell's friends and colleagues react in various amusing ways when the career-driven executive announces her unlikely desire to become a SMBC; Sloane's plot becomes complicated when she starts a comical sexual relationship with her sonographer (during a transvaginal scan no less). In *Parks and Recreation* (2009–2015) hilarity ensures when Ann Perkins decides to become a SMBC and is faced with potential sperm donors with the names Sewage Joe and The Douche (she eventually decides against the SMBC pathway entirely, not wanting to conceive a 'Little Douche').

In UK television, SMBC representation often focuses on the "seediness" of insemination. In the crime drama *Silent Witness* (2021), the SMBC storyline is associated with sordidness and corruption when an investigating officer mocks the deceased pregnant solo mother Laura for using a known sperm donor. Donor conception is further mocked when the prolific sperm donor, mockingly referred to as 'Frank the Wank', is identified as a potential assailant and as a sleazy and pitiful creature: 'Why would Laura resort to "Frank the Wank?" (Thomas 2021). In the comedy Netflix series *The Duchess*, written by and starring comedian Kathrine Ryan, donor conception is described as a shameful practice: as 'stick[ing] some pathetic random loser's spunk up yourself' (MacDonald 2020). In this limited series described by *Variety* as a 'tasteless misfire' (D'Addario 2020), the stereotypical view of the single mother is evident: 'Of course, as soon as you hear the phrase "single mother", you automatically fear the worst: DNA tests, lie detectors' (MacDonald 2020). *The Duchess* initially documents Katherine's journey to become a SMBC; however, so idealised is the co-parenting route that she eventually opts to co-parent with her criminal ex-partner despite their relationship being one of abuse in which her ex has called her: a 'cunt', 'tired old gash', and 'pathetic skank groupie' (MacDonald 2020).[3] Yet, Katherine chooses to co-parent with an abusive man she describes as 'the worst human being that I have ever met' (MacDonald 2020). Why does she choose this? Because the nuclear family co-parenting model—even when toxic and abusive—is idealised over the SMBC route.

In fact, positive portrayals of SMBC often only come in narratives in which solo motherhood is eventually abandoned and matrimony secured. The prevalence of the "happy ending" in fiction through the incorporation of the father into the family unit chimes with Juffer's claim that while single mothers may gain respect for how confidently they exercise their autonomy, 'the respect is most quickly earned if single mothers operate as if they were a nuclear family, temporarily minus the live-in-dad' (2006, 5). In these stories, not only is a happy ending obtained but respect for the single mother is more easily achieved as the romance genre implies that singledom is temporary and fixable.

However, a happy ending doesn't necessarily need to include the donor/biological father; any romantic pairing will work if it transforms the one-parent family into a co-parenting ideal. One contemporary television show which habitually enfolds single mothers into romantic relationships to indicate happiness, success, and salvation is *Workin' Moms*. I briefly mentioned this series earlier but will expand on the show's treatment of single women in more detail here. In her first episode of *Workin' Moms*, work-obsessed publishing executive Sloane describes herself as career driven and anti-relationship:

> You know I used to think there was something wrong with me. Relationships, family, the whole idea of it almost kind of bored me. I don't know. My life really took off when I started working. So I became the man I wanted to marry. (Horodyski 2021)

When Sloane decides to become a solo mother through sperm donation, her sister asks, 'Are you really ready to become a mother? I mean … what about your job? How are you going to manage all that?' Sloane replies, 'I don't know, I'll figure it out' (Staav 2022). During her pregnancy, Sloane starts dating her ultrasound technician and co-parents with him when the child is born. Sloane's return to work is only made possible through her boyfriend acting as a stay-at-home parent. Success for Sloane is that she is able to obtain the dream of "having it all": a career, a child, and a (rather submissive) romantic partner. Sloane's struggle to prioritise her child and earlier scenes in which she recklessly endangers her six-year-old niece present Sloane as someone who would have floundered as a solo parent. The introduction of a boyfriend who has no scenes independent of being Sloane's live-in childcare, works to enable Sloane to be an adequate mother and career woman.

Sloane is not *Workin' Moms* only SMBC. A solo parent journey is attempted in Season Three with Bianca. This SMBC pathway is abandoned after five episodes when Frankie confesses her love for newly pregnant Bianca. The pair instantly consummate the relationship and enfold the pregnancy within a two-parent family unit. Bianca even tells Frankie, who is a woman and lesbian, that Frankie is 'the best father Solomon [her child] could ever ask for' (Wong 2020) in an act to present the two-parent family as still male/female framed.

Beyond the solo mother pathway, *Workin' Moms* includes two single mothers, one of whom has a similar salvation storyline. Following divorce, Val is raising two teenage sons alone who disrespect and terrorise her; Val is enveloped into a romantic relationship in Season Four and it is only the presence of Val's male partner that neutralises her sons' abusive behaviours. Season Seven concludes with just one single mother represented: Jenny is a single divorcee and is the show's villain. Jenny is consistently presented as selfish, a compulsive liar, a malevolent schemer, and narcissist who is unfaithful in relationships and a dangerously negligent mother. The message unfortunately seems to be that good women find partners whereas toxic characters like Jenny remain single.

All that said, *Workin' Moms* has some moments of positivity surrounding donor conception. One notable scene features Sloane's boyfriend Paul stating that he is donor-conceived and reassuring Sloane that donor babies 'have the best moms' (Horodyski 2022a). However, Sloane herself has misgivings about her pathway, confessing that her reluctance to share her pregnancy news is because she thinks it proves her to be 'feeble, imbalanced, unreliable, temperamental' (Horodyski 2022b). Moreover, solo parenthood is not presented as a positive choice and happy endings are only reached when a romantic partner is inserted. However, it is not only romance that is obtained—relationships carry a high degree of convenience. When Bianca embarks on her solo parenthood journey, she tearfully confides, 'I don't know why I thought I could do this alone' and reflects that couples have 'someone to help [them] out with everything, to carry some of the weight' (Sternberg 2019); in *Workin' Moms*, success is the achievement of a relationship that enables these moms to continue to work. Sloane, Bianca, and Val find a person to 'carry the weight' and while these arrangements are couched as love these women have also found co-parenting relationships that facilitate a full-time career. In fact, shortly after having Solomon, Bianca leaves her baby with her new partner, Frankie, and absconds on a work trip and never returns to the screen. The fact that Jenny does not find anyone to 'share the weight' is presented as a fitting punishment for her undesirable personality traits. Jenny's single status problematises her ability to hold down a permanent job and she becomes caught in a hopeless loop of trying to entrap men to validate her existence.

When Juffer optimistically states that, in comparison with historic treatment, today 'Single moms aren't immediate objects of shame and exclusion' (2006, 15), the word 'immediate' is key. As evidenced in the above examples from *Workin' Moms*, the initial presentation of solo/single motherhood is neither shaming nor problematic. However, as the storylines progress it becomes clear that a more ideal parenting model is that of co-parenting and this model is quickly and successfully adopted. Jenny, the problematic narcissist, is the only remaining single mother and is largely excluded from the central mothering clique; her actions, mothering style, and personality are certainly presented as shameful. So, while single mothers are not immediately presented as objects of 'shame and exclusion' in the series *Workin' Moms*, this is ultimately what unfolds over the seasons.

Shame and exclusion can also be internalised. In the short fiction story *What to Expect* by Robin Romm (2015), the impulse decision to become a SMBC and procure donor sperm haunts the overwrought protagonist, Emily, who agonises over the impracticality of her decision and attempts to overcome her problematic circumstance by attaching herself to a love interest. Emily's quest for romance with Elliot Green positions the heterosexual romantic fantasy as the protagonist's priority with her pregnancy demoted to a hollow subplot. While Emily's donor-conceived pregnancy is written as anomalous, her romantic obsession is written as natural and primal; when Emily encounters Elliot, who is a married man, she experiences 'That animal sense when alone with an attractive man' (Romm 2015, 115). In fact, the following description replaces the traditional depiction of the growing foetus blossoming within the uterus with the significance of Emily's romantic relationship with Elliot:

> She felt it growing inside her—the swelling affection, the manic attention to his texts. When he got near her, every cell in her body leaped up and stood erect, the hair on her arms, even the hair on her neck. A baby grew inside her, too, nurtured, she thought, by this twin affection. (Romm 2015, 122–3)

The growing baby has a secondary impact on her body and is twinned now with her gestating affections for Elliot; her love interest is now responsible for the 'swell' and genetic infusement ('every cell in her body leaped'). The protagonist effectively amputates the donor from her pregnancy narrative and presents the child as emerging after her physical union with Elliot. She reconceives her child and her use of a donor becomes an inconvenient footnote to a story on solo motherhood by choice ironically entitled *What to Expect*. The twinning of pregnancy and romance reconstitutes the twinning of lover and mother and in turn the god/goddess binary. When Emily attempts to assign agency to the foetus it is purely in the interest of retaining the affections of Elliot who may exit the burgeoning relationship: 'She imagined what the baby might say if it could speak through the placenta, uterus, muscle, and skin. The baby's words would be *stay, stay, stay*' (Romm 2015, 124). Repetition becomes a familiar device to replace the thudding of the foetus' heartbeat with the mantra 'Elliot, Elliot, Elliot' (Romm 2015, 125). Emily's story ends with the breakdown of her romance and the loss of Elliot causes her to spiral through a series of devastating questions: 'Who would love her now? What had she done to herself? How had she so irrevocably messed up her life?' (Romm 2015, 129). Emily is thus presented as chaotic and ruined without a male partner. The destruction of her relationship with Elliot comes when he decides to remain with his wife, Belle, with whom he parents a baby conceived with the same donor sperm as Emily's foetus. Elliot chooses to remain committed to the nuclear ideal and Emily is positioned as abandoned by the only chance she has at legitimising her pregnancy; as she reflects in the final sentences of the short story: 'She hadn't intended to live this way' (Romm 2015, 130).

One novel that quite literally portrays a love interest saving the "fallen goddess" is C. L. Howland's novel *The Good Life* (2019). In this novel, Madison is a SMBC who unknowingly conceives with illegally procured sperm. Unbeknownst to Madison, her sperm donor is male celebrity Ring Stanford who had his sperm stolen following medical rape. Ring finds out about the illegal harvesting and selling of his sperm and seeks out Madison with the intent of claiming his unborn child. After an explosive meeting between Madison and Ring, a romance ultimately ensues, and the donor-conceived child is born to into a heteronormative traditional family structure. The novel is packed with typical romance tropes including Ring catching Madison when she trips and falls while heavily pregnant.

What is interesting about Howland's novel is the interplay between Madison buying sperm and Ring's feeling of ownership over the pregnancy. Ring's early obsession with taking the baby from the mother positions Madison as a surrogate and the repetitive reference to 'my child' identifies the baby as a possession that he subsequently attempts to procure. Essentially the attempt by Ring to purchase the baby levels the playing field, so to speak, neutralising any accusation that Madison paying for gametes was immoral. In their transactional approach to pregnancy, they are apparently 'equal'. The addition of love to the plot works to smooth over any issue of contract and both Ring and Madison are saved from their "sins of transaction" by birthing the child into a traditional family structure. The plot advocates for known biological parentage; Ring criticises Madison for choosing the 'unknown' (anonymous donor conception) and Madison explains that she chose against adoption because she wanted a blood connection to the baby (Howland 2019, 35). Rather than her pregnancy representing the strength of choice, Madison is written as weak and vulnerable; she blames moments of emotional fragility on 'hormones' and her status as a single woman is described like poverty: 'How long has it been since someone had asked if I was warm enough? A very long time' (Howland 2019, 70, 72). When the pregnancy and Ring and Madison's romantic relationship is leaked to the media, the headline 'LOVE CHILD' works implicitly to suggest that a child not conceived in a relationship is not a product of love (Howland 2019, 133). The male protagonist's name, "Ring", obviously symbolises the importance of commitment and traditional family values—an extended metaphor that is realised in the novel's conclusion when the couple marry and the baby is born into a family with two biological parents.

In *Single Mother: The Emergence of the Domestic Intellectual*, Juffer makes the following salient point about legitimisation:

> [S]ingle mothers who make it clear that they want some day to remarry are "eligible for future legitimacy" and thus granted temporary respect and even admiration. By contrast, single mothers who work to construct alternative and long-standing family formations and who construct a political and social identity around single mothering as a preferred status represent a less legitimate, although perhaps not completely illegitimate, position. (2006, 17)

I suggest that the "leniency" we witness in fiction, in which a character has the potential for future legitimacy (Sloane, Bianca, Madison), is not shared with characters like Romm's Emily and *Workin' Moms'* Jenny because they are depicted as undesirable and therefore not likely to secure future legitimacy. Both are consequently written off as not deserving respect nor admiration.

The drive to secure legitimacy is so important in fiction featuring solo parents that Nelson found that sexual intercourse is used as a plot device to validate conception in Hollywood films featuring sperm donation. Nelson notes that while sperm donation may happen within the plot, 'it really takes sex—ideally sex accompanied by romantic love—to make a family' (2014, 60). Nelson identifies that in most romantic comedies featuring sperm donation, a heterosexual romance effectively erases the role of donation in the narrative. In the films *The Switch* (2010), and *The Backup Plan* (2010), a happy ending is achieved when a man becomes part of the family unit. Indeed, if we look at advertisements for the film *The Backup Plan* (2010) posters read 'Fall in love. Get married. Have a baby. Not necessarily in that order'. A pink arrow suggests that, in this film, having a baby comes first but love should come next and then marriage. This not only legitimises the offspring but envelops the SMBC, Zoe, back into the goddess fold as a wife. The tagline referencing love, marriage, and baby riffs off the playground 'Kissing' song: 'first comes love, then comes marriage, then comes baby in a baby carriage.' This is a preferred moral order that bioethicist David J. Velleman quips in his academic writing is 'not such a ridiculous way of doing things, is it?' (2015, 72).[4] A similar reference is made in Carol Snow's novel *What Came First* (2011)—the title of which suggests a reordering of Velleman's 'not so ridiculous way of doing things' in which the donor baby comes first and then the plot works to rectify this mistake through the protagonist's yearning for love with the donor. The plot of Snow's novel follows protagonist Laura who is a SMBC and is deliberating whether, at 40, she should attempt to provide her son, Ian, with a donor-conceived sibling. Laura breaks the rules of anonymity afforded to the donor by employing a private investigator. Once Laura meets the donor she fantasises about sexual intercourse with him and later shares his identifying information with other recipient families. This unethical act destroys the donor's life and his partner's. The unfortunate moral of Snow's story is that women desperate to have a child make reckless and selfish decisions. More troubling is that this behaviour is largely excused because Laura is simply trying to reinstate the proper order of things: love, marriage, baby—in whatever order is possible.

The legitimising of donor conception through sexual intercourse with a love interest is not a contemporary concern. In the controversial British film *A Question of Adultery* (also known as *The Case of Mrs. Loring*) from the 1950s, Mark Loring takes his wife Mary to court for divorce after she becomes pregnant with a donor-conceived child. Despite Mark agreeing to sperm donation due to his own infertility, he later changes his mind and accuses Mary of adultery. However, Mary's lawyer argues that when Mark had sexual intercourse with his wife following the donor insemination that he legitimised the pregnancy: 'Do you recall the day of May the 27th. [...] It was on that day that your wife first told you she was pregnant, shortly after you made love to her and in so doing accepted the fact of her condition. You had condoned it!' (Chaffey 1958). Although this film is not about a SMBC, it shows that from the 1950s to the present day, sexual intercourse is presented as a means through which to metaphorically erase donor conception, legitimise conception, and establish a nuclear family structure.

While I agree with Nelson that sexual intercourse is a dominant theme in donor-conception focused films, I note that in the examples I have presented here it is not only via sexual intercourse that conception is legitimised and it is not only in film we see this tendency towards legitimisation. What I call "corrective solutions" occur when the SMBC enters any sort of co-parenting relationship—it does not matter if this is heterosexual, romantic, healthy, or stable. From Katherine's choice of an abusive co-parenting arrangement over solo motherhood in *The Duchess*, to Emily's attempt to ensnare a married man during pregnancy in *What to Expect*, to Bianca's lesbian romance with Frankie in *Workin' Moms*, the examples explored here show that any coupling is preferred over solo mothering, no matter how positively solo motherhood may have initially been presented. I argue that "corrective solutions" are not about sex and heteronormativity, but are focused on solving the "problem" of single motherhood and preventing the perpetuation of the struggling solo woman who is still very much demonised in society. While a heterosexual nuclear family is preferred as the ideal structure, any co-parenting structure will do. In the stories in which solo mothers do not find a co-parenting relationship they are often villainised as reckless, negligent, and selfish—as seen in the YA literature examples discussed previously. I am reminded of the phrase "be part of the solution, not part of the problem"—the SMBC is invited to be part of the solution which is a two-parent family, or be part of a single-parent problem.[5]

In many of the fiction examples I examined, the introduction of a male partner to the SMBC narrative does two things to counteract the single woman "problem". First, the author furnishes the solo mother with the fairy-tale ending as articulated as desirable in memoirs by Jane Mattes, Genevieve Roberts, and Morrissette (explored in more detail in the next chapter). However, secondly, the addition of a male love interest also facilitates the reintroduction of what Haraway calls 'old hierarchical dominations', including heteronormative reproduction, 'Family/Market/Factory', and sex; furthermore, it re-establishes the dichotomies of male/female and god/goddess (1991, 161). The reinforcement of dichotomies is evidenced in the title music for *The Duchess* (2020) in which composer Oli Julian attempts to celebrate the strength of women but the phrase 'woman, woman, she's a lover and a mother' undermines any attempt at a feminist anthem because it intrinsically connects romance with mothering and positions a woman as having two principal roles: sexual and nurturing.

Portraying women as either lover or mother is popular in many of the texts presented here and comes from a long history of compartmentalising women as either good or bad. This compartmentalisation has its roots in the ancient tradition of storytelling through which societal and cultural attitudes towards the "compliant" woman and the "rebellious" woman are explored through mythic tales in which those dichotomies become the characters of heroine/witch, biological mother/evil stepmother, beauty/hag, chaste/promiscuous, mother/spinster, and mistress/wife. These reductive stereotypes appear often in fairy tales—which are foundational narratives within society, offered as entertaining stories but embroiled with clear messages, warnings, and guiding themes. As English Historian Marina Warner notes, 'Fairy tale is essentially a moralizing form' (1995, 25). While many fairy tales do not feature mothers (they are often dead or have been replaced), they do feature women who exist on a sliding scale of acceptability to villainy. When Warner notes that fairy tales 'engage with issues of light and darkness' and differentiate 'normal from the monstrous' this includes how women are plotted as good or evil. The 'simplistic dualism' Warner identifies as core to the fairy tale has been 'annexed to ugly ends' and weaponised for political gain and control (1995, 410). If 'Storytelling can act as a social binding agent' (Warner 1995, 414), this can be particularly dangerous if one group receives sustained negative attention.

Unfortunately, the tales offered here—from *The Switch* to *Silent Witness* to *Headlock*—shape the myth of the SMBC in our contemporary. Such stories are fed by, and fuel, stereotypes on single and solo mothering. As Warner notes about the purpose of fairy tales:

> The tale must sense the aspirations and prejudices, the fears and hunger of its audience; like seaside pier palm-readers, fairystory-tellers know that a

tale, if it is to enthral, must move the listeners to pleasure, laughter or tears; if they fail in this, nobody will want to hear their stories anymore. (1995, 409)

Stories like *The Duchess*, through its confrontational nature and timely connection to ongoing debates in society over the acceptability of donor conception, will be remembered diversely by those who are entertained by the plot, those who enjoy the comedy, those who dislike the crudeness, and those who disagree with the content. In essence, the negative portrayal of the solo mother via gamete donation reflects 'the aspirations and prejudices' of its audience. Unfortunately, these narratives, through vast societal reach, can become a primary way for the public to learn about donor conception and solo parenthood.

In the next chapter, I will explore memoir writing by SMBC. Many "Plan B" SMBC articulate in their memoirs that they struggled with abandoning the fairy-tale "happily ever after" that involves creating a family with a lover or spouse. In these stories, the SMBC mourn the death of the lifestyle they desired—that of a romantic partner with whom to conceive and raise children. However, although there is a sense of loss associated with needing to (temporarily perhaps) proceed solo, these narratives resist suggestions that choosing to be a SMBC was spontaneous, reckless, regretted, and a rash act of selfishness. It is possible, we find in memoir, to find strength in compromise and to find that while romance might have been a preferred route, it is not presented as a "fix" for a "problem" lifestyle. Furthermore, even for the Plan A mother who may not feel a fairy-tale loss, the problem of the fairy tale still exists because if matrimony has not been secured by the "good" woman, the only other role in this polarising space is to default to the "bad" witch/hag/promiscuous/spinster/mistress role that has been demonised since early mythic tales.

Conclusion: What Is To Be Done?

The literary examples presented in this chapter act to hold the cyborg mother back in a binary system and this is an act of erasure for those who identify as something other than heterosexual, coupled, and/or sexually inclined. In Mieko Kawakami's novel *Breasts and Eggs* Kawakami provides one of the more thorough and sincere explorations of the donor conception pathway in fiction.

SMBC Natsuko first discusses her intent to become a SMBC with Jun, a donor-conceived adult; her choice to speak directly to a donor-conceived person implies that the ethical debate surrounding conception must prioritise the voices of those directly involved. Jun and his friend Yuriko explain their trauma at discovering later in life that they are donor-conceived which helps Natsuko to conclude that the 'problem' with donor conception is 'the lying and coverup' and ongoing stigmatisation of the pathway that leads to a desire for subterfuge (Kawakami 2020, 236). Reflecting on the "selfishness" of reproduction itself—as I discussed in the previous chapter—Natsuko asks whether there is 'any form of childbirth that did not involve the egos of the parents?' (Kawakami 2020, 229). This is something Yuriko speaks about when she explains that much of her criticism directed towards donor conception is applicable to all types of reproduction—that really no one should procreate. Natsuko reflects on the testimony of those with lived experience in the donor conception community to inform her decision making. Natsuko chooses to conceive a child with Jun and raise the child with awareness of the child's origins. Kawakami's work champions donor conception using a non-anonymous donor and advocates raising children with transparency.

Despite the restrictions imposed in Japan, *Breasts and Eggs* reveals that the SMBC pathway is a real, but very underground, movement. On solo mothering, Natsuko attends talks and conferences, immerses herself in forums and blogs, and even sees a special feature on the news. Yet, women who choose this route are shamed; in the news feature on SMBC, a solo mother masks her identity and speaks of the lack of options available to a woman wishing to reproduce: 'I'm honestly still shocked I went through with it' (Kawakami 2020, 183). Natsuko finds herself with few advocates and little support for her to become a SMBC. For single mother Makiko who raised her child alone following divorce, SMBC is a 'dumb' decision because Natsuko is actively choosing single parenthood when it is heavily criticised.

Natsuko's decision to become a SMBC via sperm donation in a country that forbids it presents her as triumphantly resistant to patriarchal control. In the novel, many women are depicted as trapped under patriarchal systems: initially Natsuko believes that she must endure sex as a service to her boyfriend and Natsuko's male editor tries to restrict her creative freedom. Natsuko's married friends reflect on their feelings of powerlessness and entrapment in their marriages, with some stating that they would not wish to save their husband's life if it were endangered and others noting that they would be obliged to in order to survive: 'I need him to keep working. How could I maintain my current lifestyle if he died on me?' (Kawakami,

2020, 152–3). This conversation draws attention to the dominance of nuclear family constructions and the endurance of the traditional 'ideal' in which the husband is the provider. So extreme is the plight of the woman trapped in unhappy marriages that Rie describes herself—as her mother before her—as 'free labor with a pussy' (Kawakami 2020, 251). Natsuko's decision to resist societal pressure to enter a romantic relationship which will make her unhappy, aligns powerfully with how Haraway describes the cyborg as a beacon of hope even if construed externally as an unpalatable thing: 'Cyborg unities are monstrous and illegitimate; in our present political circumstances, we could hardly hope for more potent myths for resistance and recoupling' (1991, 154). Natsuko's manipulation of the clinic sees her taking control of her body and new reproductive technologies; this chimes with Haraway's argument that '[c]yborg imagery can suggest a way out of the maze of dualisms in which we have explained our bodies and our tools to ourselves' (1991, 181). Natsuko takes the tools of assisted reproduction—IUI or IVF—and uses them to her own ends as a SMBC which not only contradicts the law in Japan but contradicts the dualism inherent in much child rearing discourse as being mother/father led. However, the power of Natsuko's resistance is limited. While Natsuko manipulates the fertility clinic to secure treatment, her resistance is quiet and hidden; she must masquerade as partnered to be worthy of treatment. Even a text as progressive as *Breasts and Eggs* cannot refuse the pull back into the nuclear family ideal in the final pages. While this conclusion is not presented as a fairy-tale happy ever after for Natsuko, it is offered as the only option.

The lack of positive representation in literature, film, and television restrains the liberational SMBC path and positions it as a threat to the nuclear family tradition which is often erroneously presented as the healthier way to have offspring. Representation has not significantly improved since the demonisation of Mrs. Loring in *A Question of Adultery* which accuses fertility doctors of creating 'phantom fathers to fill the world with test tube babies' (Chaffey 1958). This is a problem. Haraway describes her Cyborg Manifesto as 'a coming to terms with the world we live in and the question "What is to be done?"' (Gane 2006). I too ask, what can be done about the lack of nuanced and positive representation for SMBC? In Kawakami's novel the answer to 'what can be done?' is openness towards donor conception and transparency over assisted reproduction. Natsuko herself holds the answer to the problem when she notes that in researching SMBC she found mainly 'memoirs or extended interviews' (Kawakami,

2020, 185). Natsuko laments that there is no other positive representation available (as evidenced in this chapter) but as Natsuko comes to learn, the most significant and important narratives are those presented by the donor conception community itself.

In the next chapter, I turn to look at how solo mothers are presenting and exploring lived experience in memoir, podcast, testimony, and interview. While it is unfortunate that popular culture is not more measured in its presentation of SMBC, I hope that the popularisation of solo mother autobiographical works will see the production of better informed and more balanced pieces in the years to come. When Haraway writes that the cyborg is 'a creature of social reality as well as a creature of fiction' (1991, 149), it should be the case with SMBC discourse that the fiction is informed by the reality. In Chap. 5, I look at the lived reality of women who have become solo mothers through gamete donation and question how we can use these materials to better inform practitioners, ethicists, and the public to ensure that 'social reality' is not lost in the shadow of "bad and sad" mothers in SMBC fiction.

Notes

1. Stories which feature both the background of donor conception and the threat of the stranger could be said to be metaphorically examining the anxiety and dangers associated with donor anonymity. *Feathered* (Kasischke 2008) is one example of this. The main plot in *Feathered* involves the disappearance of Michelle, a donor-conceived child; Michelle goes missing, and after an extensive search is discovered as an anonymous person living in a remote location. Michelle has amnesia and remembers nothing of her life. There is a clear parallel here to how the sperm donor is often written: anonymous, afar—and often—searched for. Michelle's amnesia also reflects the identity struggle some donor-conceived children face when not knowing the other half of their genetic background. Through amnesia and anonymity, the donor-conceived child and the donor become united in erasure. The message, therefore, is that anonymity is haunting and consuming.

2. Ros became pregnant following a casual relationship and chooses to proceed with the unexpected pregnancy.

3. Similar language is used to describe the villainised mythic figure of Lilith from Jewish midrash and single women like her, as articulated in the poem 'Lilith Jumps the Fence': 'They say he [Adam] invented names, and its true / He called me shrew, bitch, witch, / And dumb cunt' (Ostriker 1993, 94). It is notable that in both texts, 'cunt' is used to diminish women to genitalia which is presented as the nucleus of undesirable behaviours.

4. Reflecting on the same playground song, donor-conceived person, Kiara Schuh, notes that the song is both outdated and designed to highlight 'traditional family stereotypes' but that her solo mother benefitted from changing attitudes towards women, family, and households, which meant that by the time her mother considered parenthood 'the idea you needed a husband to financially support your family was irrelevant' (Schuh 2022, 9). This change in attitude Schuh and her mother attribute to the feminist movement, especially women who spoke out against restrictive and stereotypical ideas on marriage (2022, 11).

5. The idea of "fixing" the issue of being single is also reflected in studies, scholarship, and lived experience. In Tine Ravn's book *Lived Realities Of Solo Motherhood, Donor Conception And Medically Assisted Reproduction* she notes that SMBC may 'need to rework the order of the biographical elements, and therefore many state that a child needs to come first and then a partner may follow later on' (2021).

REFERENCES

Barnsley, N., and S. Clarkson. 2018. *Our Story: How We Became a Family.* Donor Conception Network.

Bright, K., dir. 1996. *Friends.* Season 3, episode 3, "The One with the Jam." October, 1996, on NBC.

Chaffey, D. 1958. *A Question of Adultery.* Eros Films.

Chalifour, F. 2009. *Call Me Mimi.* Toronto: Tundra Books.

D'Adamo, A.F., and E. Hoffman Baruch. 1986. Whither the Womb? Myths, Machines, and Mothers. *Frontiers: A Journal of Women Studies* 9(1): 72–79. https://doi.org/10.2307/3346135. Accessed December 3, 2023.

D'Addario, D. 2020. 'The Duchess' Is a Tasteless Misfire by Netflix: TV Review. *Variety*, September 2. https://variety.com/2020/tv/reviews/the-duchess-review-katherine-ryan-1234755496/. Accessed November 15, 2023.

Davis-Floyd, R., and J. Dumit, eds. 1998. *Cyborg Babies: From Techno-Sex to Techno-Tots.* London: Routledge.

Franklin, E. 2007. *The Other Half of Me.* London: Random House, ebook.

Gane, N. 2006. 'When We Have Never Been Human, What Is to Be Done?' Interview with Donna Haraway. *Theory, Culture & Society* 23 (7–8): 135–158. https://doi.org/10.1177/0263276406069228. Accessed December 2, 2023.

Gibson, W. 1984. *Neuromancer.* London: Gollancz.

Gill, J. 2017. *Left Out.* 13th Sign, ebook.

Haraway, D. 1991. A Cyborg Manifesto: Science, Technology, and Socialist-Feminism in the Late Twentieth Century. In *Simians, Cyborgs, and Women: The Reinvention of the Nature*, 149–182. New York: Routledge.

Hayles, N.K. 1999. *How We Became Posthuman: Virtual Bodies in Cybernetics, Literature, and Informatics.* Chicago: University of Chicago Press.

Hoffman M., and R. Asquith. 2010. *The Great Big Book of Families.* London: Francis Lincoln.

Horodyski, M., dir. 2021. *Workin' Moms.* Season 5, Episode 2, 'Mamma Mia Meatboy.' February, 2021 on Netflix.

———., dir. 2022a. *Workin' Moms.* Season 6, Episode 6, 'Oh. Ohh. Ohhh.' May, 2022 on Netflix.

———., dir. 2022b. *Workin' Moms.* Season 6, Episode 7, 'Goin Fishing.' May, 2022 on Netflix.

Howland, C.L. 2019. *The Good Life.* Random Tangent Press.

Juffer, J. 2006. *Single Mother: The Emergence of the Domestic Individual.* London: New York University Press.

Kasischke, Laura. 2008. *Feathered.* London: HarperCollins e-books.

Kawakami, M. 2020. *Breasts and Eggs.* Translated by Sam Bett and David Boyd. New York: Picador.

Landon, B. 2002. *Science Fiction After 1900: From the Steam Man to the Stars.* London: Routledge.

MacDonald, T., dir. 2020. *The Duchess.* September 2020, on Netflix.

Mattes, J. 1997. *Single Mothers by Choice: A Guidebook for Single Women Who Are Considering or Have Chosen Motherhood.* New York: Three Rivers Press.

McLoughlin, L. (2020) 2023. *You Look Like Me* podcast. https://podcasts.apple.com/gb/podcast/you-look-like-me/id1537873411. Accessed November 18, 2023.

Mendlesohn, F. 2007. Introduction. In *The Cambridge Companion to Science Fiction,* ed. Edward James and Farah Mendlesohn, 1–12. Cambridge: Cambridge University Press.

Morrissette, M. 2008. *Choosing Single Motherhood: The Thinking Woman's Guide.* New York: Houghton Mifflin Company.

Nelson, M.K. 2014. Hollywood Sperm Donors. *Contexts* 13(1): 58–60. http://www.jstor.org/stable/24710834. Accessed December 3, 2023.

———. 2019. The Presentation of Donor Conception in Young Adult Fiction. *Journal of Family Issues* 41(1): 33–61. https://doi.org/10.1177/0192513X19868751. Accessed December 2, 2023.

Ostriker, A. 1993. *Feminist Revision and the Bible.* Cambridge: Blackwell.

Parke, R.D. 2013. *Future Families: Diverse Forms, Rich Possibilities.* Oxford: John Wiley & Sons.

Parr, T. 2010. *The Family Book.* New York: Hachette.

Potter, B. (1908) 2013. *The Tale of Jemima Puddle-Duck.* London: Penguin.

Quinn, P., and K.R. Allen. 1989. Facing Challenges and Making Compromises: How Single Mothers Endure. *Family Relations* 38(4): 390–395. https://www.jstor.org/stable/585743. Accessed December 4, 2023.

Ravn, T. 2021. *Lived Realities of Solo Motherhood, Donor Conception and Medically Assisted Reproduction*. Emerald Studies in Reproduction, Culture and Society.

Roberts, G. 2019. *Going Solo: My Choice to Become a Single Mother Using a Donor*. London: Piatkus.

Romm, R. 2015. What to Expect. *The Missouri Review* 38 (2): 111–130.

Russ, J. 1974. The Image of Women in Science Fiction. *Vertex* 32 (1): 53–57.

Schuh, K.R. 2022. *Chosen Family. A Donor Conceived Woman's Journey to Redefining Family*. Amazon.

Shippey, T. 2008. Hard Reading. In *A Companion to Science Fiction*, ed. D. Seed, 11–16. Oxford: Blackwell.

Snow, C. 2011. *What Came First*. New York: Penguin.

Staav, Y., dir. 2022. *Workin' Moms*. Season 6, Episode 3, 'Bye Bye Goldie.' May, 2022 on Netflix.

Stauffacher, S. 2003. *Donuthead*. Random House.

Sternberg, P., dir. 2019. *Workin' Moms*. Season 3, Episode 4, 'Training Day.' January, 2019 on Netflix.

Sweeney, Joyce. 2006. *Headlock*. New York: Open Road, ebook.

The Donor Conceived Community. 2023. https://donorconceivedcommunity.org/. Accessed November 12, 2023.

The Donor Conception Network. 2023. The Donor Conception Network. https://dcnetwork.org/.

———. n.d. Personal Stories. https://dcnetwork.org/useful-info/personal-stories.

Thomas, D., dir. 2021. *Silent Witness*. Bad Love: Part 1. September, 2021, on BBC.

Velleman, J.D. 2015. Family History. In *Beyond Price: Essays on Birth and Death*, 1st ed., 61–78. Cambridge: Open Book Publishers. http://www.jstor.org/stable/j.ctt17w8gwg.7. Accessed March 4, 2023.

Warner, M. 1995. *From the Beast to the Blonde: One Fairy Tales and Their Tellers*. London: Vintage.

We Are Donor Conceived. 2023. https://www.wearedonorconceived.com/. Accessed November 18, 2023.

Wong, J., dir. 2020. *Workin' Moms*. Season 4, Episode 8, 'Charlie and the Weed Factory.' May, 2020 on Netflix.

CHAPTER 5

Personal Storytelling: The Solo Mother and Lived Experience

Abstract Through reflecting on personal accounts by Solo Mothers by Choice (SMBC), I explore how and why women are choosing (in the words of Genevieve Roberts) to 'go solo'. In this chapter, I also discuss the importance of storytelling in the donor conception community and how stories from lived experience can provide authentic and positive representation of the SMBC phenomenon which is either largely overlooked or demonised in contemporary culture.

Keywords Assisted reproduction • Collaborative witnessing • Family • Fairy tale • Fertility • Fiction • Gamete donation • Interview • Lived experience • Memoir • Narrative • Nuclear family • Single mother • Solo mother • Stereotype • Stigma • Storytelling

REFLECTION

> Experience exceeds the narrative, but experience can only be organized and communicated based on narrative. (de Serpa et al. 2019, 175)

On an exceptionally warm day in the first week of September, my twins' Reception[1] class teacher came to the house for an informal "meet the teacher" visit. I wore a dress (ditching my more favoured jeans and band t-shirt ensemble) and had curled my pink hair. My twins rejected the shirts and corduroy trousers I had selected and so instead of perfectly presented boys opening the door, the teacher was greeted by a monster wearing a top hat and a barefoot prince holding a hobby horse. We collectively ushered the teacher into our immaculate living room. And it was immaculate. Absolutely immaculate. A veritable show home.

I had stayed up the night before cleaning the house. I scrubbed the kitchen, washed the bed linen, dusted throughout, and vacuumed behind furniture, all for a woman who would sit on the sofa in my living room for thirty minutes. I mowed the lawn, trimmed the wisteria, and climbed up a ladder to cut back the overgrown rose arch over the door (just in case she happened to glance 8 ft up). I even reordered the bookshelves, twice. The first time I organised my books in colour order, but I didn't like the jumble of the heights, so I rearranged them in height order by theme. The week before the visit I actually repainted a wall because it looked a bit mucky (little hands like to press against pale walls), so the dining room wall got a fresh coat of Jasmine White. In hindsight this was absolute madness. Later, when I recounted the visit to a friend, she explained my actions as overcompensation: 'Us single mothers', she said, 'have to work harder; we have to fight every day to seem competent and respectable.'

The teacher was warm and friendly; she asked the boys about their interests and made notes. She asked about their likes and dislikes, whether they followed a special diet, if they had allergies, who would be collecting them from school … and so on. Then she turned to me—was there anything else I wanted her to know?

'The boys are donor-conceived; I'm a solo mother', I said. One of the boys helpfully chipped in that I had gone to London and my doctor was called Alison. I explained the reason behind this disclosure was because I'm very transparent about our family setup and also because she'll need to know this ahead of any discussion of families in class (say, on Father's Day). She nodded along happily enough, making the odd note here and there.

Before the teacher left, I gave her a Primary School Resource Pack[2] published by the Donor Conception Network. I felt embarrassed as I passed it to her. It felt like I was handing over a user manual: *this is a forty-three-page guide to my life choice*. I tried to excuse the whole awkward affair by clumsily telling her that she didn't have to really look at it if she didn't want to. She flicked through it as I attempted to indirectly apologise for inconveniencing her with paper:

'You might find the information on language important—we use donor, not father or daddy; there are also some suggestions on books for the school library. I don't know if it'll be useful but …'

'Thank you. Stories are important', she said.

I, a literature scholar, believe that to be one of the trustiest statements ever issued.

She turned to my boys and asked them if they had a favourite story. Fortunately for me they are born book lovers and have many favourites. But the reigning favourite at the time was *The Quest for a Flower Baby: A Story for Children Conceived Through Donor* by Kathryn Heffernan which reworks the idea of the traditional princess fairy tale. In Heffernan's story, the technology of donor conception is expressed through the metaphor of a princess choosing a special flower from the Field of Family so she can become a solo mother. She embarks on a quest, and traverses the darkest of forests and climbs the tallest mountain, all in an effort to become a solo mother.

Fertility treatment is often described as the Everest of reproduction. In clinics we are guided over treacherous terrain towards a summit some never reach. After eleven unsuccessful rounds of IVF, adventure activist Jessica Hepburn actually climbed Everest; scaling the world's tallest mountain only took three attempts.

But then—DRAGON.

In *The Quest for a Flower Baby*, the princess climbs her Everest and then, quite unexpectedly, she encounters a dragon: 'And just when she thought she had reached the field, a large dragon swooped down from the sky. He said, "You cannot pass"' (Heffernan and Edwards n.d., 9).

The climb is hard and we know it will be hard but no one anticipates the dragon at the top. The dragon can be many things: an anomalous test result, failed implantation, or unviable pregnancy. The dragon appears just when you think everything is going your way—just when you approach the summit of Everest.

My dragon was thyroid disease. A diagnosis that was a shock because, until that point, I thought my only barrier to conception was my lack of sperm. So, I embarked on another climb—this a literal one. I scaled London's Shard (via lift!) to meet my second consultant, a doctor called Alison Taylor. In Chap. 2, I mentioned this journey and how I travelled in silence while overlooking the city.

Rather than feel small and insignificant overlooking the sprawling metropolis, I felt massive; I felt that my desperation to be a mother dwarfed London and that this consultation was the most important moment in the world. In the waiting room, I felt uncomfortably expansive, like I was sucking the air out of the clinic. The seat felt too small, I felt too big, the air felt too hot, and the time ticked too slowly. I pulled at my collar, and I felt an urge to run—not away from the situation but deeper into it. I wanted the consultation now, the answers now, the procedure now, the baby now; because with every tick of the clock I imagined my fertility decaying.

Alison helped me fight the dragon, assisted by the magic of levothyroxine. Once the dragon was vanquished, my story concluded with my finding two babies in the "Field of Family". My twins. Me, a mother at last. A happy ending.

Thinking back to the day we welcomed the teacher into the house, I see now that what I was trying to do was tell her a story. From the painted wall to the DCN school pack, I was trying to tell a story. A story of many chapters—celebratory, explanatory, but also defensive.

In this chapter I think about the SMBC and the importance of personal storytelling.

Introduction: Real Experiences

In the last chapter I identified dominant fiction narratives which present the solo mother as an ambitious career woman, reckless deviant, or struggling single woman. Invariably, the solo mother—successful or otherwise—is portrayed as finding happiness only in romance. This is an old issue and connects with how women have been linked to stereotypes in ancient goddess mythology (see Chap. 2 and the work of Bolen 1984). When Donna Haraway says she would 'rather be cyborg than a goddess', she chooses to push against the restraints imposed by mythic understandings of what a woman is; and, in choosing to be a SMBC, many women are saying the same (1991, 181). So far, I have drawn attention to the many ways in which the cyborg helps to reframe what reproduction and family can be despite the prioritisation of the nuclear family historically, in anti-donation discourse, in clinical spaces, and in fiction. However, what has yet to be explored are the actual real-world experiences of the mothers I have been discussing. Throughout this book, I have discussed the ways in which the cyborg represents new language, new social reality, and a struggle for meaning. I now turn to look at how SMBC use personal storytelling to articulate a new social reality of family and how, through narrative, SMBC explore the complexities of what it means to be solo by choice.

In Haraway's 'Cyborg Manifesto', she writes that '[s]ocial reality is lived social relations, our most important political construction, a world-changing fiction' (1991, 159). In citing the cyborg as a 'world-changing fiction', she too reflects on the significance of storytelling for imagining new possibilities. As I noted in the last chapter, there is a tendency to connect the cyborg to science fiction and Haraway also does this when she identifies science fiction writers as 'theorists for cyborgs' because their work challenges social and physical boundaries. For Haraway, science fiction writers are 'story-tellers exploring what it means to be embodied in high-tech worlds'; however, I argue that SMBC also explore 'what it means to be embodied in high-tech worlds' by narrating how it feels to use assistive technologies to conceive beyond the traditional boundaries of the nuclear family setup (Haraway 1991, 173). I suggest that through lived experience storytelling, the personal SMBC narrative emerges as "world-changing non-fiction". However, to truly be world-changing the dominant narratives of single mother disadvantage, selfishness, and threat to nuclear idealism need to be transformed. This is a big and ongoing task but one that is already underway in SMBC memoir. Following on from the previous chapter in which I showed how fictional stories can be reductive and damaging in the ways that they perpetuate stigma and ideals, here I pivot on the concept of storytelling and think about how narratives of lived experience have the power to be positively transformative through their potential to defend, clarify, and educate.[3]

When I speak of "narratives of lived experience" and "lived experience storytelling" (terms I use synonymously), I refer to the range of ways in which SMBC relay information and explain their experiences about being solo parents through gamete donation. These stories may be offered through published memoir, informative guides, and podcasts and interviews; they may be recorded online in support forums, expressed in community meetings (both formally and informally), and offered casually to friends, family, and acquaintances. The stories they offer in informal and formal contexts are a way to celebrate, normalise and destigmatise the decision to become solo mothers. In doing this work they also empower their offspring to know that their family structure is one to be respected rather than hidden. By sharing their stories, SMBC rehumanise the cyborg by elevating the discussion from external spaces (e.g. moral debates and fiction) to provide an insight into the internal issues, struggles, and decisions of choosing gamete donation.

Beyond examining the real experiences of SMBC, this chapter delves into the importance of lived experience storytelling in the donor conception community. The UK's Donor Conception Network (DCN) places enormous emphasis on sharing stories of donor conception (see Pettle and Burns, n.d., 15). The DCN hopes to not only diversify how conception is taught to young people but to normalise this diversity. Their *Telling and Talking* series (Montuschi 2013) includes guides, booklets, and pamphlets aimed at sharing the donor story with colleagues, teachers, friends, and family members, and their *Our Story* (Barnsley and Clarkson 2018) series is aimed at children and depicts different types of conception journeys (including sperm donation, egg donation, double donation, embryo donation, and surrogacy). Here, I explore how lived experience storytelling helps provide a positive representation of SMBC and challenges the stigma and stereotyping associated with this family structure and conception pathway. Helping me tell these stories are nine participants who volunteered to discuss their experiences of being SMBC. I am grateful to the following women, all friends of mine who have been such a large part of my own journey as a mother, who contributed their lived experience to this chapter: Alexis, Eleni, Michelle, Nicola, Sam, Sarah A, Sarah B, Tamara, and Victoria.[4] The purpose in this chapter is not to critique these biographical accounts or provide an overview of everyone's experiences—but instead to explore some of the shared themes in these pieces and how community-based storytelling presents opportunities for education. I will start by looking at how some solo mothers articulate the complexity of what it means to "choose" donor conception and then discuss how the voices of SMBC can be used to tackle lingering misconceptions.

CHOICE, FAIRY TALES, AND PLANNING FAMILIES

In this section, I will provide an overview of how some SMBC discuss the tricky issue of choice. In the last chapter I exposed how, in fiction, embarking on solo parenthood is often framed as a "bad choice". This "bad choice" is highlighted in numerous ways from the regretful solo mother (Romm's *What to Expect* 2015) to the angry and hurting donor-conceived child (Sweeney's *Headlock* 2006). The issue of choice is also a strong theme in most guides and memoirs on SMBC. Unlike many fiction texts suggesting that the decision to parent solo is a rather fun and impulsive act (e.g. Franklin's *The Other Half of Me* 2007 and Chalifour's *Call Me Mimi* 2009), many stories about lived experience identify the solo motherhood pathway as a time-consuming and difficult decision to make.

In Mikki Morrissette's *Choosing Single Motherhood* chapter 'Grieving the Childhood Dream', she explains that '[s]ingle motherhood can feel like a decision of "no other choice" rather than of choice' (2008, 43). This position resonates with Tine Ravn, who writes that single women choose solo motherhood because

> they have not found the right partner with whom to have a child as a result of various factors, and their great desire to experience motherhood and concerns about increasing age and fertility decline motivate them to initiate treatment before it is 'too late' for them to have a child of their own. (2021)

This was the case for Liv Thorne who begins her memoir, *Alone*, with a note regarding the loss of her 'naive fantasies' about romance with the line, 'I'm not going to lie, I didn't ever dream it would be like this' (2021, 1). The issue of no choice is partly rooted in the fact that many women feel a loss of a wanted co-parenting romantic partner. In many memoirs this is coded as the loss of the fairy-tale happily ever after or the ending of a dream.

In Jane Mattes' memoir *Single Mothers By Choice*, she suggests that most women dream of marriage: 'To be happy being an SMC [single mother by choice] you need to come to terms with giving up your dream' (1997, 4). Likewise, in *Going Solo*, solo mother Genevieve Roberts reflects that '[b]ecoming a solo parent is not my fairy-tale wish' (2019, 36). In the introduction to the podcast *No need for Prince Charming*, host Alisha Burns, a SMBC, addresses the SMBC community and assumes that '[i]t never crossed your mind that Prince Charming wouldn't come along' (Burns 2022a). The loss of a traditional happy ending was mentioned in many of the interviews I conducted.[5] For example, Michelle notes that being a solo mother was not her original plan for family construction: 'In an ideal world I'd have met the right person to start a family with and live happily ever after.'

Frequent references to fairy tales and princes underscore how the "failure" to achieve romantic coupling is connected to ideas of failure as women and mothers. The Disneyfication of optimal womanhood and motherhood is not limited to fantastical narratives of princesses securing matrimony (*Snow White* 1937, *Cinderella* 1950, *Sleeping Beauty* 1959, *Beauty and the Beast* 1991), but a wider issue of how the advertisement of marriage as an achievement is so ubiquitous.[6] Sarah Thompson in *Happy Single Mother* explains that 'our cultural obsession with the nuclear family—at best a Disney-esque concept, rooted in religion and fuelled by a wildly out-of-control wedding industry—makes us blind to the many possibilities and opportunities that an alternative approach can bring' (2023, 7). Bearing this in mind, Morrissette's articulation of the longing for The One gains greater significance when she writes that she not only missed a having a spouse but the pageantry involved in marriage: 'giving up the traditional childhood dream of a glorious wedding followed by babies can be very difficult' (2008, 43).[7] In 'Episode 3' of her podcast *Single Mother by Choice*, Emilia Thompson notes that young people are conditioned to believe that 'you cannot simply be happy unless you are in a relationship or unless you're married' (2022). In an interview with me, Nicola articulates concern over how the conditioning of fairy-tale ideals can harm reproductive decision making. Nicola explains that because she 'grew up on Disney movies and fairy-tale endings', there was an expectation of partnership which was not only presented as guaranteed but as the key to happiness. Nicola points out that the conditioning of girls and women to need a partner for validation is pervasive:

> It's not just Disney or other movies/tv that condition us to believe in the 2.4 future. It's just life. The number of times I got asked if I had a boyfriend throughout my life is amazing. It's almost like you're defined by who you're dating.

For Nicola, choosing to be a SMBC was not easy, and it took her five years to be comfortable with her decision to embark on solo motherhood through donation.[8] Nicola explains that she needed to give herself time to adjust to a new vision of the future and a new way of imagining what her family would be like: 'I always thought I'd find "the one"; deciding to "go solo" was a difficult decision to make.' In hindsight, Nicola notes that the promise of a perfect partner and the social pressure to achieve romantic fulfilment made becoming a SMBC harder to accept long after she had made the decision.

It is in narratives which express longing for, and bereavement toward, the loss of the fairy-tale promise, that we see the more complex treatment of what choice motherhood means. In these accounts, many women articulate that SMBC had become the only option after the dream of romantically informed co-parenting had to be retired (although sometimes temporarily). It is in these discussions that what I have been calling "Plan B" is often articulated. This means that there was originally a preference not to be a SMBC and the decision to pursue solo parenting became necessary due to pressure stemming from age and fertility. When Ravn notes that 'the break between real and ideal causes ambivalence and reveals a paradoxical feature of the "choice" of embarking upon solo motherhood', she identifies the contradiction of the Disneyfication of family (real v ideal) and the ironic concept of choice (to make a choice when there is no other option) (2021). Again, there is a dualistic element to the "problem" here in which both a partner and a baby are desired but may not coincide; and waiting for a partner may mean giving up on motherhood entirely.

The issue of waiting can be a major factor for those pursuing SMBC; how long does a woman wait for the "dream" before embarking on solo motherhood? Sometimes the wait is described as not being long enough. For example, in the fiction of the previous chapter many romantic "happily ever afters" are achieved after donor conception has been sought—often during pregnancy (e.g. *Workin' Moms*) or soon after (Howland's *The Good Life* 2019). These examples suggest that seeking donation was rash and that waiting for a partner would have been prudent. Yet many SMBC describe waiting for a long time and, in some cases, taking years to start treatment. For Sarah B, she waited until the point at which waiting longer would have jeopardised her chances of motherhood; she chose the solo route despite initially struggling with the decision to conceive using donor sperm: 'If it was not due to my age I likely would have delayed this longer; although now I have my daughter I wish I had done it many years ago.' In Nicola's case, it took her seven years to finish her conception journey; during this time Nicola endured medical complications, operations, many rounds of IVF, numerous embryo transfers, and two miscarriages before finally completing her family of three with the arrival of two girls. When she mentions that the journey was 'hard and tiring and there were times when I really didn't want to do any more injections', it is difficult to identify the SMBC route as an impulsive act. Waiting for years and undergoing complex processes to create a family is not uncommon. From starting the journey to giving birth, it took Sam five years. Likewise, Eleni underwent five IUI treatments and three rounds of IVF, relating that the entire process made her feel 'completely broken'. Becoming a SMBC is never described as a rash action by the mothers themselves.[9]

So far, I have discussed the complexity of choice. I mentioned how for some SMBC becoming a solo parent was not the first plan for family construction. However, for some women like me, conceiving through donation to create a one-parent family was a first choice; this is sometimes articulated as Plan A. When I talk about Plan A, I understand this to mean solo motherhood through gamete donation as the first choice for family planning. Plan A is often connected to people who do not want a romantic partner and/or a co-parent.[10] When Susan Golombok et al. in their 2021 study 'Single Mothers by Choice' write that '[s]ince the 1980s, a growing number of single heterosexual women have made an active decision to parent alone and have had children through donor insemination', they overlook the wealth of SMBC who are not single nor heterosexual.[11]

Yet, is separating out SMBC as either Plan A or Plan B helpful? Or is it just another dualism that needs disrupting? The availability of assisted reproduction, donor gametes, and the freedom of women to pursue both independently unites all SMBC as exercising agency. In Mikki Morrissette's memoir she reflects on how a friend spoke of Morrissette's 'courage' at becoming a solo mother, and this is true regardless as to how and why the SMBC pathway was chosen. Louise Sloane, author of *Knock Yourself Up*, notes that there are many reasons a woman might choose donor conception but whether Plan A or Plan B, 'having the child was the non-negotiable part of the equation' (2007, xi).

In the interviews I conducted, many participants discussed how their plans for a family evolved over the years. Victoria notes how her main goal was always motherhood: 'I didn't want to risk not having a child and family of my own so my Plan A [marriage first, then children] became Plan B to go about having my own family solo.' Likewise, for Alexis, despite originally intending to co-parent with a partner, she identifies solo parenting as a Plan A because the main objective was to become a mother; the mode through which this was pursued changed. Alexis says: 'I have always felt comfortable knowing I was going to bring children up by myself [...] I tried to find the traditional expected way of finding someone. Always knowing if it didn't happen, I would go down the solo route.' Michelle makes a similar point when she notes that 'Plan B became Plan A'; although Michelle originally wanted the traditional "happily ever after" of marriage and a nuclear family, the adjustment of her plan was not something that caused her distress. Michelle explains that the option of becoming a solo mother was one she welcomed: 'I was quite comfortable with using a sperm donor, excited perhaps.' Years after completing her family, Michelle reflects that she is content with solo motherhood: 'I am not "grieving" for a life I could have had, or wishing I'd taken another path. I love my life, grateful for being a solo mum, with no "husband" issues.' Sarah A not only spoke about the malleability of plans but that different life stages involve different priorities: 'Now I am happy as a single woman. I feel more like I have made a Plan A in my post-45 years as I now know what I need and feel empowered over my own life.'

In many cases the option to pursue solo motherhood through gamete donation was considered to be a practical and positive option while other avenues (such as co-parenting) were first explored. Eleni notes that becoming a solo mother by choice was one option in the overall plan to become a mother: 'I wanted to be a mother and that was my plan. I had always been open since my 20s to achieving that in whatever way possible. I always felt comfortable exploring the option of being a solo mum.' Similarly, Sam identifies the fluidity of choice and adapting what 'Plan A' means based on circumstances:

> Solo motherhood had always been an option for me. Ideally, would I have a partner to help me out? Sure that would be nice, but it definitely wasn't "the be all and end all". I was approved as a solo adopter way before I looked into donor conception, so it has definitely never been a Plan B option.

Sam, as a member of the LGBTQ+ community, knew she would always need donor gametes if she wanted to have biological children and so the distinction between Plans A and B was never clear because even if co-parenting was a desire, gamete donation was always required.

The issue of choice for the solo mother is complex and unique to each individual. In all examples presented here, unlike the representation in popular culture, making the decision is often articulated as a slow and considered journey. The study by Elia Psouni, Julia Berg and Hanna Persson found that the solo mothers they interviewed all wanted to 'present themselves as strong and competent' (2022, 1). Yet, they note that there is a 'struggle for recognition as responsible, stable parents, and a frustration over repeatedly having to defend and justify their choices' (Psouni et al., 2022, 1). Likewise, in the 2021 pilot study of solo women undergoing assisted reproduction in Demark, it was found that although their SMBC subjects did not identify with narratives of vulnerability, they needed to be ready to defend their choice to become solo mothers due to societal stigma (Steenberg et al. 2021). However, for others, as is the case with Michelle, she found strength and confidence in choosing to be a solo mother and, in her experience, has not encountered a need to defend her lifestyle: 'I was always confident around my life choices; comfortable with the decision I'd made, open about it to friends, even work colleagues. No particular challenges around it at all, and I was always met with positive responses—to this day, I've never had a negative comment.' This is why storytelling is so important. Through lived experience storytelling the act of defending and justifying can be made easier through providing testimony to challenge inaccurate and inappropriate fiction narratives and anti-donation discourse that dominate social and cultural understandings of non-traditional lifestyle choices.

Guides, Educating, and Collaborating

So far, I have provided a brief overview of how lived experience narrative has the power to clarify misunderstood issues by looking at one frequently discussed topic: choice. Over the last few chapters, we have seen how clinics perhaps do not represent choices for solo parenting as well as they could; we have seen how anti-donation discourse suggests that donor conception is a bad choice; and we have seen how reproductive choice outside of marriage is considered reckless in fiction. Lived experience narrative provides real, practical, and helpful stories of how difficult it can be to choose gamete donation. In this section, I want to push further and look at how SMBC lived experience narrative educates formally (through publications) but also informally through the casual sharing of personal experience in day-to-day life. Here I examine three main ways SMBC use their voices to educate others. First, I will look at how SMBC recommend choosing solo parenting over "settling" for an inadequate relationship; then I consider how SMBC offer an education on different options for family construction, and finally I discuss how these shared experiences underscore the importance of transparency and openness in the donor conception community.

In many lived experience stories, SMBC explain solo parenting as a more sensible and rational pathway than settling for a romantic or co-parenting relationship that might be damaging or problematic. While anti-donation ethicists like David J. Velleman and 'Feminist Against Progress' Mary Harrington would argue that solo parenting is damaging, what SMBC experience shows us is that the most stable environment is one in which the parent feels safe, fulfilled, and happy. Yet, for Harrington, "settling" is a sensible approach. Harrington suggests avoiding the trappings of searching for 'Big Romance' and instead recommends making strategic decisions on partnering. Often, there are claims that SMBC are picky (supported by popular news reports that SMBC chose donor conception because "Mr Right" had not come along). Harrington speaks of the "plight" of women overlooking potential partners because they do not want to "settle". She writes that there are 'ever-escalating expectations for how perfectly their partner should match' and a want to 'marry up' meaning that many good men are 'written off as potential partners' (2023a, 92–3). However, some women do not want a man (I am one of them). Some women do not want a relationship (I am one of them). These women have the right to avoid problematic relationships, and they have the right to avoid caving to social convention and peer pressure to fulfil a nuclear ideal. Harrington goes as far as to say that 'if you're among the great majority who wants kids, you're better off getting married—that is, by definition, "settling"', but also claims that she is not suggesting everyone gets married or stays in abusive relationships (2023a, 185). Yet, her following line seems to connect motherhood to a relationship: 'There have always been women who don't want to be mothers, who don't want relationships with men, or who don't want relationships full stop' (2023a, 185). By making motherhood seemingly dependent on heterosexual marriage there is the implication that women should settle for men, unsuitable relationships, and sex—even if they do not want to—to become parents.[12] 'More freedom', Harrington writes, 'doesn't always equal more happiness' (2023a, 187). But it can.

In interviews with SMBC such a pragmatic approach to relationships is considered damaging and instead solo mothers recommend taking a different approach to finding stability by conceiving and rearing solo. Speaking to Burns in her podcast, interviewee Rachel explains that her success as a mother comes from not settling for an unsuitable partner just to adhere to social expectations: 'being a solo mum makes me a much better mother than I would have been if I had been in a relationship' (in Burns 2022d). Rachel's advice to the listening audience is, 'You don't need to tolerate another person's behaviour to have a baby one day. Only be in a relationship if it makes you primarily happy and enriches your life' (in Burns 2022f). Likewise, in conversation with SMBC life coach Mel Johnson, Genevieve Roberts (who later does happily marry, years after becoming a SMBC) notes that she embarked on solo motherhood because she felt that her previous relationships were not stable enough for children and that she did not want to settle (Johnson 2020). For Roberts, waiting to 'get it right' was the most sensible thing to do, but she could not wait to get pregnant—a woman's fertility does not wait kindly. Sarah A recounts a similar encounter when she describes one of her friends gently encouraging her to pursue the solo pathway: 'A defining moment in the decision was really when talking to a dear friend about wanting a partner to give the child stability. She said, "But surely the most stable situation is to be alone?"'

The cyborg is not an 'all-out war on relationships' as Harrington fears (2023a, 71) but instead marks a space for new relationships to form. The cyborg represents the freedom to not have to choose a relationship, and to refuse ill-fitting ones. Prioritising children over romance does not mean the termination of a romantic future. In *Knock Yourself Up: A Tell All Guide to Becoming a Single Mom* (2007), Sloane's 'girlfriend's guide' to becoming a solo mother makes the point that while many women reject 'the idea of getting into a bad marriage, or the wrong marriage' they are not rejecting marriage, romance, or men; instead they are making a judgement call at the time in which compromise with an unsuitable partner is not wise. In her introduction, Sloane states that unfortunately the idea that '[s]ingle moms can be great moms' still reads like an 'apparently controversial' statement (2007, xii). Sloane, a SMBC, concludes that '[b]eing raised by a good single mom is a lot better than being brought up inside a bad marriage. Love makes a family' (2007, xi). Her advice is succinct but powerful: 'quality beats quantity when parents are concerned' (2007, xiii).

Another driving factor behind SMBC storytelling is the importance to communicate options to women for alternate routes to reproduction. In Burns' podcast, it is clear that many women did not realise that solo motherhood was a viable option. Rachel, in episode fifteen, notes that she did not realise SMBC was a viable pathway: 'If I had known that there were women actually doing this, I would have done it ten years earlier' (in Burns 2022e). Rachel explains that she tried to make relationships work but now understands that co-parenting was not the right path for her: 'I really tried hard to do the nuclear family thing but it just was never for me; and I knew that so long ago but I just didn't realise there were other alternatives that were normal' (in Burns 2022e). In terms of school education in the UK, interviewee Tamara notes that 'I definitely don't think parenthood by gamete donation is discussed enough if at all in education.' Eleni similarly comments that she does not feel that solo motherhood via gamete donation is 'clearly presented or discussed anywhere' and as a result, 'it is still not seen as "the norm" and there is a lack of understanding and information.' So much focus is placed on contraception in secondary school education that women are unaware of fertility and infertility issues and options. Sarah A explains that her experience of school sex education was limited to the repeated warning of 'don't get pregnant'. Victoria notes how options for reproduction were not clear to her and that early education is key to ensuring that young people not only know routes available to them in terms of family construction but also have a better understanding of their own reproductive systems:

> I wasn't actually aware of it [SMBC] as even an option, and not sure how I came across it to be honest. […] But then I don't think family planning is properly discussed either. We are told about how not to get pregnant. But not informed about the "body clock" fully, such as egg quality decreasing with age, options to freeze eggs and embryos. The awareness needs to be presented and discussed much much earlier so we are better informed and can make some decisions potentially earlier.

Arguably, testimony offered by SMBC bridges the gulf that exists between school education on reproduction and the reality of the diversity of family construction pathways.

However, not all tools of education are framed positively. Some SMBC non-fiction texts inadvertently contribute to the unhelpful and unfortunate stereotype that the single mother is a mother who struggles financially, emotionally, socially, professionally, and often psychologically. Books like *Accidentally on Purpose: The True Tale of a Happy Single Mother* (Pols 2009), by title alone, suggest that happiness for the single mother is anomalous, so much so that a book claiming to connect happiness and single parenting must boast of its surprising authenticity. Even books designed for inclusion can be positioned unhelpfully; the title of Nancy E. Dowd's *In Defense of Single-Parent Families*—albeit unintentionally—presents the single-parent as needing rescue, support, and understanding. Many self-help books use their titles to offer hope and suggest that the guide can help single women find happiness, thereby (perhaps indirectly) implying that happiness is not easily located in single motherhood and needs to be sought after, fought for, and achieved: Nicole Elizabeth Biggs, *The Single Mother's Journey To Wholeness: Hope And Help For Single Moms*

(2005); Maria Roberts' memoir *Single Mother on the Verge* (2009); Amy Rose and Emma Cotterill's *Surviving Solo Motherhood* (2022); and, Sarah Thompson's *Happy Single Mother: Real advice on how to stay sane and why things are better than you think* (2023).

In Rebecca Cox and Zoe Desmond's *How to be a Happy Single Parent* (2023), they aim their text at four types of single parent: separated parents (e.g., divorcee), unintended single parents (e.g., unplanned pregnancy without a partner), solo parent by choice (e.g., by adoption or gamete donation), and widows. Here, one-parent families are described as united together and collectively striving 'to be good parents to happy children'; the book is designed to help one-parent families negotiate a 'society built for two-person parenting teams' (Cox and Desmond 2023, 10). The strength of such an approach is the establishment of commonality and therefore community; however, like many support texts that have come before, the focus on helping the reader to achieve happiness—while certainly useful to some and benevolent at heart—continues to position one-parent families as bound up in sadness. There remains little representation for individuals who have confidently and happily chosen solo parenting as their primary pathway (or new plan) for family construction. There is nothing wrong with these books, or their approaches and titles—and I do not wish to deny that solo motherhood can be challenging—however, these titles do reveal that single/solo motherhood is often marketed through its association with challenge rather than success. A cursory walk through a bookshop, or a casual online book search, will paint a certain picture of what contemporary single motherhood looks like that it is not altogether positive. While the adage is true—"never judge a book by the cover"—sometimes that first impression is the one that resonates.

That said, there are some positively positioned texts such as Emma Johnson's *The Kickass Single Mom: Be Financially Independent, Discover Your Sexiest Self, and Raise Fabulous, Happy Children* (2017). Further, it should be noted that despite the more problematic titles, these texts offer uplifting stories of growth, strength, and perseverance. Importantly, the popularity of these guides to single/solo motherhood and their availability in mainstream bookshops demonstrate public and academic interest in this type of parenting and family dynamic. Problematic titles aside, there is a spirit of cooperation and support at the heart of this movement. Professor of Philosophy and Women's Studies, Naomi Scheman is right when she notes that the increasing numbers of women choosing single/solo motherhood means that 'it's entering the realm where it gets talked about, written about' (cited in Renvoize 2023). The growing wealth of guides shows not only the importance of storytelling, but the necessity for storytelling to educate.

Nevertheless, formal storytelling through guides, and informal storytelling offered day to day by SMBC sharing their experiences either with friends and acquaintances or in forums and podcasts, highlights how important transparency is today for families who have chosen gamete donation. The need for transparency adheres to donor conception industry recommendations and is sensitive to the advice of donor-conceived people. Furthermore, through transparency it is communicated that SMBC is a positive pathway rather than something associated with secrecy and embarrassment. In conversation with me, Nicola notes the multilayered importance of storytelling in her own life. Nicola describes how the explanation of her conception pathway leads to personal empowerment, meaningful engagement with others, and a sense of normalcy for her children:

> I was initially concerned about people's opinions of me. At some point I accepted that I had no control over what others thought, but could control what I thought and felt. I've actually found the more confidently I talk about having used a donor, the more comfortable people seem to be talking about it. I've had many "that's what I would have done if I hadn't met my partner" and several "I wish I'd done that" from divorced women. I am completely comfortable with my decision now and will happily talk about it to others. I feel it's important for me to talk confidently about my decision to use a donor, as I don't ever want my children to feel anything but confident about their origins.

In the above example Nicola describes an informal scenario in which she is open to unplanned conversations with a range of people. Genevieve Roberts, author of *Going Solo*, like Nicola, speaks about the importance of openness as connected to communicating positivity around the choice to become a SMBC: 'If I was going to do this, I was going to do it and be proud of it, I mean I've written a book about it' (in Johnson 2020). As a journalist by trade, Roberts found a public and formal space in which to professionally and personally share her story and experience. Simultaneously, informal localised discussions (casual conversation) and formal broader sharing (memoir) contribute to the drive for education and openness and, in doing so, tackle misunderstandings, stigma, and sensationalism rife in many of the dominant narratives that have been covered in this book.[13]

In mainstream UK media there is increasing interest in how celebrities are creating their families using assisted reproductive technologies, namely surrogates and sperm donors. There is a notable difference in how celebrity SMBC are discussed in comparison to non-celebrity women. I will take the case of singer-songwriter Natalie Imbruglia, who conceived a child through IVF and sperm donation in 2019 as one example. The newspapers *The Mirror*, *The Sun*, and *The Independent* all reported the news neutrally but only cited positive Twitter (now X) comments and used language like 'showed off' and 'cute' to describe the baby. Imbruglia's announcement inspired news articles on SMBC in which women shared their journey to solo motherhood using sperm donation. For example, an article in *The Sun* cites Imbruglia's pregnancy announcement and notes that 'increasing numbers of women' are intentionally pursuing motherhood without a partner (Clarke and Culley 2019). This article includes three mothers but is skewed with sensationalist reporting as it includes a description of a SMBC having conceived through a 'one night stand'. In reality, the mother conceived during a short-term casual relationship; the biological father knew of the pregnancy and opted not to co-parent. Other articles use more damning language, drawing attention to implied recklessness and danger; for example, in 2022 *The Sun* ran the headline: '"MIRACLE BABY" I had sex with the world's most famous sperm donor to fulfil my dream of motherhood' (Rogers and Cleave 2022). *The Daily Mail* covered the same story with the addition of the words 'notorious sperm donor' and 'desperate for a baby' (Brennan 2022). Other articles draw on spontaneity and rash decision making through using descriptions like this: 'one day [she] woke up set on becoming a mother' (Wade-Palmer 2023).

Nicola reflects on how SMBC reporting is often unhelpfully skewed:

> I do not feel that solo motherhood is considered to be a mainstream method of parenthood, although it is being discussed more and more. It helps that several celebrities have said they have either considered, tried or actually used this route to parenthood. Solo motherhood has been discussed on several talk shows, but sadly the emphasis is often on the type of donor used (unregulated internet donors), rather than going via a clinic/sperm bank, presumably to create sensationalist headlines.

Genevieve Roberts has featured in a range of positive pieces of SMBC journalism, some of which she has authored, such as 'A mother's story: I had two babies with a sperm donor—then I found love' (Roberts 2022).

Roberts, a journalist, is better positioned to negotiate the news media industry than some individuals who become prey to the more predatory tabloids. Positive representation is more likely to occur when the interviewee has a degree of control over the narrative. In the case of Roberts, more nuanced and positive portrayals of SMBC come from working collaboratively with the press with which she has authorial presence.

In the article 'Between Perspectives: Narratives, Lived Experience, and Culture' (2019), Octavio Domont de Serpa Jr et al. discuss the importance of 'collaborative witnessing', which is a useful concept to think about in terms of how diverse narratives can, and should, converge. So far, many of the dominant narratives on SMBC are siloed from autography; in this chapter I have shown through memoir and interview how many of the negative assumptions and arguments made about SMBC in anti-donation debate and popular culture texts are not reflective of real experience. Collaborative witnessing is a practice in which lived experience is 'written in a joint way with a researcher' to inform 'care and knowledge production' in the interests of valuing and learning from experiences beyond the institution; in doing so, collaborative witnessing can be therapeutic and lead to meaningful and positive change in attitudes and care towards community groups (de Serpa et al. 2019, 174). de Serpa et al. acknowledge that this form of collaboration is important because of the differences inherent in how experience comes with different types of power and knowledge dynamics (2019, 174). This is certainly the case with hierarchical consultations in clinical spaces in which communities are advised in a top-down approach, but the same communities are not consulted as to what the best care and practice is for them. de Serpa et al. articulate the importance of testimony to ensure difference is identified and supported rather than smothered, 'which presupposes tolerance and the inclusion of difference, instead of its extinction' (2019, 174). Here, I suggest an opening up of what "researcher" can mean to include any party who is offering a reading of the SMBC community (whether this be the ethicist, film maker, or clinical policy maker) and suggest collaboration with their human subject.

While lived experience narratives are not to be interpreted as collective truth nor community fact, they are important narratives which articulate unique knowledge and involvement with a range of scenarios that form a tapestry of what it means to be both a patient and member of a community. Collaborative witnessing forms a vital connection between practitioner, academic, and community. This collaboration is essential when dominant narratives in popular culture can be skewed and contribute to a negative framing of SMBC in society. Slowly, there is evidence of increased collaborative witnessing. The booklet *Independent Family Planning: Choosing Solo Motherhood through Gamete Donation. A guide for fertility healthcare professionals* is written by a team of members from the SMBC community (including myself) and in consultation with Bourne Hall fertility clinic and the Donor Conception Network (Halden et al. 2023). This booklet, which has been shared with fertility clinics across the UK, highlights to industry professionals the lived experiences of solo mothers at the stages of family planning, donor gamete selection, embarking on the conception journey, pregnancy, and birth.[14]

When de Serpa et al. state that '[e]xperience exceeds the narrative, but experience can only be organized and communicated based on narrative' (175), they suggest that narrativisation of experiences is not only important but arguably the only way to meaningfully communicate. There are many studies exploring the data surrounding single/solo motherhood (the most recent report from the HFEA[15] shows a 44% increase in treatment for single people in the UK between 2019 and 2021 (Human Fertilisation and Embryology Authority 2023); however, data is just one part of the story and it is only through prioritising the lived experiences of the people to which the data relates can we start to understand the nuances, complexities, and truths of the SMBC community. It will always be impossible to conclusively and thoroughly present the varied experiences of solo motherhood, but in sharing individual stories across platforms—memoir, podcast, blog, magazine (etc.)—there is hope that negatively skewed narratives can be challenged.

CONCLUSION: THEORISTS FOR CYBORGS

The power of storytelling is immeasurable. The ways in which stories can be told are unlimited. In this chapter I have highlighted the ways in which SMBC narrativise their own experiences to guide, educate and support other solo parents, and also to challenge the stigmatisation that has long haunted all one-parent families. We can also see that by looking at lived experience, the nebulous (often sensationalist) anxieties articulated over cyborg conception are unfounded. Children are not disadvantaged, women are not casting men aside as irrelevant, and the nuclear family is not under threat. What we see in these real stories is not the cyberpunk dystopia that is commonly associated with the cyborg but the utopian stirrings of what is possible for new family formations. I am reminded of N. Katherine Hayles who notes that when agency is prioritised the posthuman is more likely to be accepted, but when agency is under threat the posthuman can be rejected (1999, 279). These real-life stories highlight individual agency and prioritise choosing the best pathway for family construction. While previous chapters have shown that assisted reproduction and donor conception can provoke anger and fear because they seemingly "disappear" and "devalue" traditional concepts of conception, we see through the testimony of SMBC the vital *appearance* and *opportunity* that come with opening up what family means.

Wherever one stands on the moral spectrum regarding what makes a normal/ethical/optimal/ideal family, the fact is that new family forms and new conception pathways exist. Listening to the stories of donor-conceived families is key to understanding this phenomenon. In terms of the families shaped by cyborg conception, by listening to their stories we can identify technical ways to improve systems, processes and treatment. By amplifying these voices, we can raise awareness of non-typical reproduction pathways which can impact policy and lead to better funding opportunities. Moreover, we can improve how donor-assisted families are viewed, received, and discussed within the influential fields of academia, and popular culture.

More locally, we might also think about the issue of language—that of how solo and single mothers are, like the goddess and cyborg, 'bound in a spiral dance' (to use Haraway's phrase, 1991, 181). In many of the memoir and guides referenced here there is slippage between whether solo or single is used to refer to the SMBC. Morrissette's book's title uses the term 'single motherhood' whereas Robert's *Going Solo* prefers the term solo mum throughout. Why is this significant? How language is used directly impacts how stories are shaped and understood. Ross Parke notes that increasingly 'single mothers' are categorised as 'poor' and SMBC are classed as 'a new group' (2013, 71). Moreover, often solo mothers are described as being more mature (Morrissette 2008, 99), better educated, and more financially secure (Bock 2000) than single mothers. In differentiating the "old group" from the "new group", is there a risk of constructing an unhelpful new dualism, that of single/solo? Worse, is the new dualism combative? Single *versus* solo.

Notes

1. First (non-compulsory) year of primary school in the UK (children join at the age of 4).
2. Produced by the Donor Conception Network in 2018 and funded by the Van Neste foundation.
3. It is important to appreciate that providing stories of lived experience will inevitably mean including others. This is something Bob Cowser Jr., Leila Philip and Natalia Rachel Singer note in 'Aftershocks of Memoir' (2011, 145). For the SMBC this not only means relating a story that includes one's children but their extended families, friends and even the donor and their families too.
4. Interviews were conducted by Grace Halden. Participants completed written interviews in October and November 2023. All interviews were conducted with ethics approval from Birkbeck College, University of London. All participants previewed and approved the use of their data in the chapter prior to publication.
5. Interviewees also addressed the loss of other more traditional routes to conception, such as using donor eggs when the initial plan and hope was to use their own eggs.
6. In Lucy Knisley's *Kid Gloves*, she explains how 'The late eighties and early nineties were a hotbed of media fascination with pregnancy and babies. This fascination persists to this day' (2019, 35). Knisley notes popular films including *She's Having a Baby* (1988), *Look Who's Talking* (1989), and *Nine Months* (1995). For many of the solo mothers interviewed and cited here, the popularity and volume of baby-focused films in the 80s and 90s may have contributed to the message that success and happiness is connected to romance and co-parenting.
7. Allan Hanson notes a connection between donor and lover for heterosexual women: 'Some single women choose as donors the type of man they might have married, and some imagine their donors as lovers and husbands. A fertility counsellor told me of a woman, for example, who fantasized that she and her sperm donor met after her baby was born, fell in love, married, and raised their child' (2001, 305).
8. In total, Nicola took twelve years to complete her family from the date she first decided to consider solo parenthood.
9. This is also the case for 'DIY' unregulated/informal donations in which a known donor is located online. While this pathway is not recommended by the HFEA due to inherent risks to the recipient, the process of locating a donor and agreeing terms is not a quick nor spontaneous process.
10. There are numerous reasons for this including (but not limited to) sexuality (e.g., asexuality) or a wish to keep dating separate from parenting.

11. In Burns' podcast she shares the stories of Australian solo mothers by choice including single lesbians and heterosexual women who simply did not want a partner or had prioritised children over romance (see Burns 2022b). Burns interviews Sal who discovered later in life that she was a lesbian and that her previous 'anti-kid' stance was due to not wanting children with a man (in Burns 2022c). Like Charlotte's story as cited by Renvoize relays, being on one's own is not always a narrative of sacrifice or loss: 'I'm not a lesbian single mother because I was never terribly whole-heartedly lesbian, and I think that has something to do with my feeling that I'm perfectly all right on my own with my baby, and that I've never had a terribly strong desire to live with a man' (2023).

12. Sex is not the "be all and end all"—not for life, romance, or baby making. Harrington laments that '[a] growing subset of young men and women are simply abandoning the field of sex altogether: a recent study shows young men and women in their early twenties today are two and a half times more likely than Gen Xers to be abstinent' (2023a, 103). For Harrington this risks not only reproduction but 'the bond between mother and baby' (2023a, 103). It is ok to not want sex (as many Plan A women will tell us), it is ok to refuse it, and it is ok to want it and pursue it. A minority not wanting sex does not asexualise the majority and it does not jeopardise reproduction, the future of the species, or complicate the relationship between parent and child. What it does is make space for different types of sex, a more diverse future for the human species, and enable new types of parenting models to develop. The emergence of new forms does not eradicate existing ones—we can coexist.

13. It is common to see published memoirs offered by writers with related career experience: journalism, publishing, and academia. It is also important to think about how funding grants (which allow research and further exploration of experience) are reserved for the academic community or for charity groups. The way in which lived experience becomes subject to hier-archisation is something Jijian Voronka reflects on when arguing that caution is needed to avoid replicating narratives which lead to dominance by a particular group (2016, 197). It is worth remembering here how studies tend to lean on SMBC narratives issued by white, middle-class women.

14. How exactly collaboration can be facilitated is what is challenging. The SMBC community boasts a wealth of important lived experience narratives from podcasts to memoir, but how can these creators ensure their voices are being heard in the influential areas of clinical care, media representation, and popular culture? Often there is a separation of narratives: clinical narratives offer a top down approach in which expertise informs care down onto the patient; testimony offers a bottom-up approach in which lived experience is offered up to help inform fellow community members and

practitioners (often in the form of guides and support texts); and media/ popular culture offer a range of narratives (often conflicting and sometimes reductive) horizontally across a vast array of interested parties (e.g. cinema audiences). How can we unite these narratives collaboratively? Finding and capitalising on opportunities to consult is one way to take action. I have included an example of how collaboration and consultation can inform practice by referencing the booklet *Independent Family Planning: Choosing Solo Motherhood through Gamete Donation. A guide for fertility healthcare professionals* published in 2023. Although I secured the funding with The Wellcome Trust, the booklet was designed by, and written by, a team of members from the SMBC community (Genevieve Roberts, whom I mentioned in this chapter, was part of this working group). Digital and hard copies were sent to fertility clinics across the UK without charge. Now all private fertility clinics have a copy of this community-led booklet and can (and hopefully will) reflect on the lived experiences presented to them when thinking about patient care, policy, marketing, and treatment.

15. 2021 data published in 2023.

References

Barnsley, N., and S. Clarkson. 2018. *Our Story*. Donor Conception Network.

Biggs, N.E. 2005. *The Single Mother's Journey to Wholeness: Hope and Help for Single Moms*. Lincoln: iUniverse.

Bock, J.D. 2000. Doing the Right Thing? Single Mothers by Choice and the Struggle for Legitimacy. *Gender and Society* 14(1): 62–86. http://www.jstor.org/stable/190422. Accessed March 4, 2021.

Bolen, J.S. 1984. *Goddesses in Everywoman: A New Psychology of Women*. New York: HarperPerennial.

Brennan, S. 2022. I Was So Desperate for a Baby I Had Sex with the World's Most Notorious Sperm Donor—And It Worked! *Mail Online*, November 28. https://www.dailymail.co.uk/femail/article-11477053/I-sex-worlds-notorious-sperm-donor.html. Accessed November 15, 2023.

Burns, A. 2022a. Introduction. *No Need for Prince Charming* Podcast. February 26.

———. 2022b. S1:E13. Carly, Lucy, Theo and Gracie. *No Need for Prince Charming* Podcast. May 23.

———. 2022c. S1:E35. Sal, Edie and Hendrix. *No Need for Prince Charming* Podcast. October 24.

———. 2022d. Bonus Episode: Mother's Day Reflections. *No Need for Prince Charming* Podcast. May 6.

———. 2022e. S1:E15. Rachel and Arlo. *No Need for Prince Charming* Podcast. June 6.

———. 2022f. Bonus Episode 4: Reflections and Advice. *No Need for Prince Charming* Podcast. December 2.

Chalifour, F. 2009. *Call me Mimi.* Toronto: Tundra Books.

Clarke, L., and G. Culley. 2019. GO IT ALONE We Chose to Become Single Mums Like Natalie Imbruglia Instead of Waiting Around for Mr. Right. *The Sun*, July 25. https://www.thesun.co.uk/fabulous/4132323/these-women-chose-to-be-single-mums/. Accessed November 15, 2023.

Cowser, B., Jr., L. Philip, and N.R. Singer. 2011. Aftershocks of Memoir. *Fourth Genre: Explorations in Nonfiction* 13 (1): 145–159.

Cox, R., and Z. Desmond. 2023. *How to Be a Happy Single Parent.* London: Piatkus.

Dowd, N.E. 1997. *In Defense of Single-Parent Families.* New York: New York University Press.

Franklin, E. 2007. *The Other Half of Me.* London: Random House, Ebook.

Golombok, S., Zadeh, S., Freeman, T., Lysons, J., and Foley, S. 2021. Single Mothers by Choice: Parenting and Child Adjustment in Middle Childhood. *Journal of Family Psychology*, 35(2): 192–202. https://doi.org/10.1037/fam0000797. Accessed January 12, 2021.

Halden, G., M. Johnson, S. Kamerkar, N. Milligan, G. Roberts, and R. Ward. 2023. *Independent Family Planning: Choosing Solo Motherhood through Gamete Donation. A Guide for Fertility Healthcare Professionals.* London: Wellcome.

Hanson, F.A. 2001. Donor Insemination: Eugenic and Feminist Implications. *Medical Anthropology Quarterly* 15(3): 287–311. http://www.jstor.org/stable/649581. Accessed March 16, 2021.

Haraway, D. 1991. A Cyborg Manifesto: Science, Technology, and Socialist-Feminism in the Late Twentieth Century. In *Simians, Cyborgs, and Women: The Reinvention of the Nature*, 149–182. New York: Routledge.

Harrington, M. 2023a. *Feminism Against Progress.* Croydon: Forum.

Hayles, N.K. 1999. *How We Became Posthuman: Virtual Bodies in Cybernetics, Literature, and Informatics.* Chicago: University of Chicago Press.

Heffernan, K., and M. Edwards. n.d. *The Quest for a Flower Baby: A Story for Children Conceived Through Donor.* Germany: Amazon.

Howland, C.L. 2019. *The Good Life.* Random Tangent Press.

Human Fertilisation and Embryology Authority. 2023. Fertility Treatment 2021: Preliminary Trends and Figures. Preliminary UK Statistics for IVF and DI Treatment, Storage, and Donation. https://www.hfea.gov.uk/about-us/publications/research-and-data/fertility-treatment-2021-preliminary-trends-and-figures/. Accessed November 12, 2023.

Johnson, E. 2017. *The Kickass Single Mom: Be Financially Independent, Discover Your Sexiest Self, and Raise Fabulous, Happy Children.* New York: Penguin.

Johnson, M. 2020. Going Solo with Genevieve Roberts. *The Stork and I* Podcast. July 8.

Knisley, L. 2019. *Kid Gloves.* New York: First Second.

Mattes, J. 1997. *Single Mothers by Choice: A Guidebook for Single Women Who Are Considering or Have Chosen Motherhood.* New York: Three Rivers Press.

Montuschi, O. 2013. *Telling and Talking: Telling and Talking with Family and Friends about Donor Conception. A Guide for Parents.* DCN.

Morrissette, M. 2008. *Choosing Single Motherhood: The Thinking Woman's Guide.* New York: Houghton Mifflin Company.

Parke, R.D. 2013. *Future Families: Diverse Forms, Rich Possibilities.* Oxford: John Wiley & Sons.

Pettle, Sharon, and Jan Burns. n.d. *Choosing to Be Open about Donor Conception: The Experiences of Parents.* Donor Conception Network.

Pols, M. 2009. *Accidentally on Purpose: The True Tale of a Happy Single Mother.* Ecco Press.

Psouni, E., J. Berg, and H. Persson. 2022. 'Solo Mothers' By Choice Experiences During Pregnancy and Early Parenthood: Thoughts and Feelings Related to Maternal Health-Services. *Sexual and Reproductive Healthcare Elsevier* 33: 1–6.

Ravn, T. 2021. *Lived Realities of Solo Motherhood, Donor Conception and Medically Assisted Reproduction.* Emerald Studies in Reproduction, Culture and Society.

Renvoize, J. 2023. *Going Solo: Single Mothers by Choice.* London: Routledge.

Roberts, M. 2009. *Single Mother on the Verge.* London: Penguin.

Roberts, G. 2019. *Going Solo: My Choice to Become a Single Mother Using a Donor.* London: Piatkus.

———. 2022. A Mother's Story: I Had Two Babies with a Sperm Donor—Then I Found Love. *The Times,* December 24.

Rogers, J., and Cleave, I. 2022. 'MIRACLE BABY' I Had Sex with the World's Most Famous Sperm Donor to Fulfil My Dream of Motherhood—His Other 53 Kids Were Beautiful. *The Sun,* November 29.

Romm, R. 2015. What to Expect. *The Missouri Review* 38 (2): 111–130.

Rose, A., and E. Cotterill. 2022. *Surviving Solo Motherhood.* Welbeck Publishing Group Limited.

de Serpa, O.D., Jr., E.M. Leal, and N.M. Muñoz. 2019. Between Perspectives: Narratives, Lived Experience, and Culture. *Philosophy, Psychiatry, & Psychology* 26 (2): 173–176.

Sloane, L. 2007. *Knock Yourself Up: A Tell All Guide to Becoming a Single Mom.* New York: Penguin.

Steenberg, M.L., R. Sylvest, E. Koert, and L. Schmidt. 2021. P-472 Single Mothers By Choice—Experiences of Single Women Seeking Treatment at a Public Fertility Clinic in Denmark: A Pilot Study. *Human Reproduction* 36 (Suppl. 1). https://doi.org/10.1093/humrep/deab130.471.

Sweeney, Joyce. 2006. *Headlock.* New York: Open Road, Ebook.

Thompson, E. 2022. Episode 3. *Single Mother by Choice* Podcast. March 4.

Thompson, S. 2023. *Happy Single Mother: Real Advice on How to Stay Sane and Why Things Aren't as Bad as You Think.* Thread.

Thorne, L. 2021. *Alone: Amateur Adventures in Solo Motherhood.* London: Hodder & Stoughton.

Voronka, J. 2016. The Politics of 'people with lived experience' Experiential Authority and the Risks of Strategic Essentialism. *Philosophy, Psychiatry, & Psychology* 23 (3/4): 189–201.

Wade-Palmer, C. 2023. 'I'm a Single Mum Who Got Pregnant from Sperm I Found on Facebook. *Daily Star.* May 1.

CHAPTER 6

Conclusion

Abstract The term Solo Motherhood by Choice (SMBC) can be read as inadvertently contributing to single mother stigma; if the solo mother has a choice, it is suggested that the single mother has none. By studying the difference between the words "single" and "solo", I will illustrate how the term "single mother" has been used historically to denote worthlessness whereas "solo" has been associated with skill. How can language be used to describe solo mother families without stigmatising other women?

Keywords Cyborg • Family • Language • Gamete donation • Single mother • Solo mother • Stereotype • Stigma • Storytelling • Terminology

Introduction: Cyborg Language

In this final chapter, I want to explore why adopting the words "choice" and "solo" has become an important linguistic decision taken by many SMBC. At the start of this book, I stated that initially it is necessary to differentiate between the single and solo mother due to the different treatment of these two distinct—but interconnected—family formations across critical and popular cultural narratives. I also explained that the words "solo" and "choice" are tricky terms that need further scrutiny. In

© The Author(s), under exclusive license to Springer Nature
Switzerland AG 2024
G. Halden, *Cyborg Conception*,
https://doi.org/10.1007/978-3-031-59386-4_6

this chapter that scrutiny will happen. First, I want to make a point about how the idea of the cyborg has impacted language. Historically, human reproduction has traditional expectations and biological certainties (male/female heterosexual sexual intercourse) which have been expressed through language as "normal" and "natural". In everyday linguistic expression, society often defines this "natural" and "normal" process as defining what family is: male/female with one or more biological children. The SMBC, as cyborg, not only marks a further shift in how reproduction can be assisted, but has an ironic language of reproduction as a solo endeavour that disrupts previous presumptions about sexuality, sexual activity, and co-parenting that traditionally underpinned language on human reproduction.

Throughout this book, we have seen examples in which language is under pressure and not able to adequately describe or define nuanced experience in terms of mediated reproduction. For example, the word "choice" is used as an abbreviation in the title SMBC, but "choice" is actually a very loaded and complex notion. The wooliness of language is also highlighted in *Cyborg Babies* (1998) when Robbie Davis-Floyd and Joseph Dumit highlight the ambiguity of choice that comes with any form of assisted reproduction. They suggest that infertile individuals may feel obligated to pursue treatment simply because it exists. Today, I think choice is more complicated, certainly in respects to the cyborg and the SMBC. First, I would suggest that being cyborg today is not something we choose but something we are, whether through conception or being born into a highly technologised world. Second, in contrast to Davis-Floyd and Dumit, I do not see reproductive technologies as simply assisting traditional reproduction but as a tool to further open up—and actualise—new ways of making babies and families. Davis-Floyd and Dumit suggest that the availability of reproductive technologies pushes 'defective body-machines, infertile women' to seek medical/technological assistance (1998, 7). However, the choice afforded by the evolution of the cyborg in combination with reproductive technologies is that even fertile "non-defective" body-machines can select alternate routes to family construction—this offers significant choice to people not enfolded into the "norm" of wanting or having heterosexual intercourse. Although intended to be liberational, one of the inherent problems with the commonly accepted term SMBC is the linguistic implication that solo women choose to be a one-parent family but (in contrast) single women do not. In the book's introduction, I flagged that, despite differentiation between single mothers by circumstance and solo mothers by choice, both types of one-parent families are united on a spectrum of selfishness. Throughout this book, it has become clear that the issues of choice and circumstance are more complex than the designation Solo Mother by Choice suggests. I have shown how in a diversity of narratives the one-parent family (regardless of choice or circumstance) is presented as problematic and prone to demonisation and even sanitisation (the correction of one-parent problem families through the establishment of the more "ideal" nuclear family). Now, in my concluding remarks, I will consider how the word "single" has been used historically to denote weakness and worthlessness whereas the word "solo" has been associated with skill and precision (e.g. to perform a solo). I will question whether this separation of terms risks a hierarchical positioning of solo mothers as superior to single mothers. How can language be used to clearly describe the uniqueness of donor-assisted one-parent families without stigmatising other women and other family forms? Although it is not my intention to conclude this book by suggesting a language overhaul, I do want to identify in this final chapter the influence terminology has not only to define circumstances but also to unite and divide communities.

Single, Solo, and Choice: A Language of Difference

The working group for the booklet *Independent Family Planning* (Halden et al. 2023) was comprised of solo parents and those on the solo-parent pathway (undergoing treatment). The working group's objective was to produce a booklet that would help articulate the SMBC patient experience to inform treatment practices and policy formation in fertility clinics. The booklet was subject to peer review and was assessed by six experts in the field including community members, academics, medical professionals, and a team from the Donor Conception Network. Support for the booklet was extremely strong; however, almost every reviewer commented on the issue of language:

- *Solo or single?*
- *What does it mean to be a 'choice' mother? Does the word 'choice' for solo mothers suggest that single mothers have not chosen to mother?*

The working group reconvened to discuss the problem of language and the wildly differing peer review reports on the matter. It became clear that there was a lack of consensus on whether the words "single" and "choice" were suitable terms because some group members were not single and some members did not want to be defined by relationship status (which "single" seems to imply more so than "solo"). Additionally, some queried the term "choice" and articulated that the word suggested that other mothers had not chosen to parent and therefore the word could be diminishing to others. Eventually, it was decided that the uniting element that bound the group together was not the slippery issue of choice and relationship status, it was the pathway—that of parenting solo through gamete donation. However, the Donor Conception Network (correctly) pointed out that changing Solo Mother by Choice to Solo Parent via Donation would be hard to establish because SMBC is the understood and accepted term within the community and has been for decades.

As stated at the start of this book, the popularisation of the term SMBC is rooted in the 1980s when Jane Mattes established the organisation Single Mothers by Choice (then abbreviated as SMC). However, Mattes, too, struggled with terminology. She wrote in her memoir that settling on an appropriate term was tricky and that the single mother by choice designation was developed to distinguish choice from circumstance:

> One of our lengthiest discussions involved what we should name the organization. We felt strongly that we wanted the name to clearly convey that it was our choice and our decision to become single mothers, unlike divorced or widowed mothers. (Some of us made the choice before conceiving, and some, like me, decided after having conceived, but we all chose motherhood at some point.) There was no name that slid trippingly across the tongue, but we finally settled on "Single Mothers by Choice" as the one that best described us: single women who chose to become mothers; single mothers who are mature and responsible and who feel empowered rather than victimized. (Mattes 1997, xxi)

Mattes had been looking into solo parent adopting when she became pregnant by a lover who decided not to co-parent. Mattes is an interesting figure because although associated with the designation SMBC and gamete donation, Mattes conceived in a more traditional way. Mattes clarifies in her definition that '[a] single mother by choice is a woman who starts out raising her child without a partner' (1997, 4) and therefore is separated from those linked to matrimony (widows and divorcees). Yet, in the course of researching for the booklet *Independent Family Planning*, I met with SMBC who were not romantically single but embarking on parenthood solo, women who were solo mothers but later married, divorcees, and widows who chose SMBC after losing their partner, and women who strongly felt that becoming a SMBC was a last resort and not a choice they wanted to make. Many support groups for SMBC use the term "solo": Solo Mothers By Choice UK; Solo Mums' Support; and Solo Parents By Choice. Mel Johnson's *The Stork and I* offers support events using the term solo (such as Thriving Solo and Building Solo Parent Resilience). When given the choice between single mother or solo mother, all interviewees for this book stipulated that the preferred term for themselves is solo. Ultimately, the working group for *Independent Family Planning* decided that while SMBC needed to be used for consistency, the word solo would be used instead of single as a term preferred by much of the SMBC community. This preference, though, is not just to mark an alternate pathway to conception (because the addition of gamete donation would do that) but to try to create distance from the stigma society continues to forge around the single mother.

In writings offered about single mothers and SMBC, the differentiation is often problematically polarised. As briefly noted in the previous chapter, Ross Parke notes, 'single mothers' are often categorised as 'poor' and they are contrasted with SMBC as 'a new group' (2013, 71). The reference to the 'new group' separates SMBC from the 'poor single mother' narrative purely through the addition of the noun 'choice'. For Sarah Hayford and Karen Guzzo, SMBC has become an 'archetype' which has been 'contrasted with other stereotypes of unmarried mothers—reckless teens with unplanned pregnancies and "welfare mothers" who have children without being able to provide for them' (2015, 72). By classifying solo as distinct from "other" unmarried mothers the very issue of choice becomes flattened out so much so that it becomes meaningless. As Hayford and Guzzo note, by positioning SMBC as something individuals choose, we lose understanding of social issues that contribute to, and shape, the wide variety of one-parent families and their complex and varied economic, psychological, environmental, and lifestyle challenges (2015, 72). While I disagree that SMBC are painted positively in the media wholesale (see previous chapter), Hayford and Guzzo make a good point that, when compared with solo mothers, single mothers are more negatively framed (2015, 72). The contrast of single and solo mothers is often made through reference to sweeping generalisations. Solo mothers are 'older' (Morrissette 2008, 99), educated and financially secure (Bock 2000), and single and heterosexual (Golombok et al. 2021). Thompson identifies that there is a different way of thinking about and speaking about single and solo mothers: 'I feel a bit envious of the "solo mum" and "by choice" monikers; they sound more empowered' (2023, 3).

In her critical analysis of Mattes memoir, Katherine Mack notes that SMBC have become a mark of 'specific and privileged class, racial, gender, and sexual location' (Mack 2020, 297). It is true that formal donation and fertility access is often beyond the reach of some, but the SMBC pathway has slowly been transforming. While Naomi Cahn's observation in the early 2000s that fertility funding is reserved for couples is still largely unchanged, it is no longer the case that assisted reproduction 'allows only rich white women to bear biological children' (2009, 8). Increasingly, younger women faced with the knowledge that egg freezing is not the solution they were led to believe[1] are choosing to become SMBC earlier on in life. The increasing popularity of informal donations means that becoming a SMBC is more financially viable. However, the demonisation of any single parenting dynamic means that, as Jane Juffer notes, despite the '[n]ew possibilities for mothering without men' solo women continue to struggle due to neoliberal processes and policies that made 'life increasingly difficult for many single mothers', whether they are single by choice or circumstance (2006, 4). As evidenced in this book, SMBC are not immune from criticism in bioethics and popular culture and are not necessarily welcomed into clinical spaces even as consumers. Juffer wonders how SMBC can 'step outside the traditional gendered and sexual expectations for raising sons and daughters'; she asks, 'how does one carry through on these possibilities?' (2006, 176). I suggest one way to step outside is to do what the cyborg does, and to move beyond restrictive binaries. Mainly, these binaries seem to operate around ideas of natural/unnatural and organic/technological; however, it now becomes clear that the terms "single" and "solo" also work as opposing states. "Single/solo" is united only through the universality of their criticism—that they are shared emblems of a "problematic" fractured family.

Language is important.[2] There is a reason why differentiation happens and why there are distinct narratives for solo motherhood by choice and single mothers. As Juffer notes, 'How one becomes a single mom shapes life as a single mom' (2006, 31) and this is especially true when the distinction can articulate unique issues related to each family formation. Single mothers will usually know the identity of their child's biological father and in most cases have some sort of support, whether this be through a custody arrangement or financial agreement; a single mother will often engage with the biological father's extended family; a single mother will often have experienced a relationship separation and will be dealing with the outcome of that. In contrast, a SMBC may not know the identity of the biological father; a SMBC may have used a known, anonymous, or ID-release gamete donor all of which come with very specific rules on contact information; a SMBC (unless they have used a known donor with which they have an arrangement or co-parenting dynamic) will not have custody or contact arrangements and no extended family on the paternal side. The distinction between these two family types prevents the conflation of two different experiences of motherhood.

For some the differentiation is stark and involves a SMBC 'taking the initiative and deliberately planning to become a single mother' (Hayford and Guzzo 2015, 71). Yet, this "taking of initiative" is not a factor that distinguishes SMBC from the anti-single parent discourse around "dysfunctionality" which has historically hounded single mothers. Not only is Jane D. Bock right when she argues that 'these "new" single mothers inherit the stigma of their poorer younger sisters' (2000, 63), but also that SMBC are often demonised as narcissistically and selfishly sacrificing the opportunity to create a traditional family in favour of preserving dangerously fierce independence to the detriment of their offspring. The problem of choice here is underscored by Susanna Graham's survey of solo motherhood which found that many SMBC worried not about the 'departure from the nuclear family per se' but rather the fact that they were '*knowingly* departing from this idealized family at the outset' (2018, 254). So, while there are narratives of SMBC privilege, the SMBC is also enveloped in the "bad procreator" debate in which they become the unfortunate and selfish spinster counterpart to the unwed and pitiful single mother. In short, if the single woman is viewed historically and socially as a failure to herself and society, then the SMBC is seen as choosing failure from the outset. Astutely, Sarah Thompson writes, 'however we arrive at our single mother status, the one thing that binds us is that we still seem to have an image problem' (2023, 4). In this respect the designations "single mother" and "solo mother" are pitted against each other but the arena in which they "duke it out" is one in which there is no winner.

Juffer asks what can be done about the stigmatisation of the term single mother:

> Can the conditions under which certain single mothers are accepted be turned, reimagined, reconceived, and transformed so that all single mothers—indeed all mothers—are supported in caring for themselves and their children, thus leading to the growth of family structures that represent true alternatives to the traditional nuclear family and its predictable gendered and sexual roles? (2006, 6)

Perhaps there needs to be a more careful application of language. By examining the early use of the terms single and solo, it is clear that even on a linguistic level there are deep divides in which one term is framed more negatively than the other. The first known use of 'single' in written English was around 1340 in fiction letters between Alexander the Great and King Dindimus by an unknown author (*OED*, s.v. "single"). The use of 'single' features in Alexander Fragment B in a plot which concerns a letter written to Alexander attempting to dissuade his army from attacking a people who live naked in caves and defenceless without any wealth. The line reads, 'We ben sengle of us silf, & semen ful bare, Nouht welde we now.' Roughly translated, the line says that the people are 'single by ourselves' and are utterly alone; they report that they have nothing and Alexander will gain nothing by attacking them. They also note that if the army comes they'll hide ('hid in oure holis').[3] In this early example, the adjective 'single' denotes weakness, vulnerability, and worthlessness. The 'single' people are no better in a group because they are 'single by ourselves'. They are also described in very different ways to the people Alexander would have been used to: the nakedness of the people suggests both poverty and a lack of modesty. In terms of dictionary definition, this history led to the development of the description single to mean 'alone, solitary' and 'unaccompanied or unsupported' (*OED*, s.v. "single").[4]

Much later, in 1695, the word solo was used by British playwright and poet William Congreve in the farcical comedy *Love for Love* (*OED*, s.v. "solo"). The primary usage is to note performance (e.g. music). Jeremy, a servant to the principal character of Valentine, remarks, 'I have a reasonable good ear, sir, as to jigs and country dances, and the like; I don't much matter your solos or sonatas, they give me the spleen' (Congreve (1695) 2010, 33). Although Jeremy is not a fan of solos (they give him the 'spleen', which means to be annoyed/angry), he uses the word solo to refer to music performed by one musician. Interestingly, a similar phrase 'solos and sonatas' was used by Sir Richard Steele in *Tatler* (1710) in a piece of journalism about 'nocturnal expeditions'—chiefly the playing of music in the street to galvanise lovers; Steele notes that this romantic pastime is popular in Italy. Steele speaks of the serenade: 'The Italian soothes his mistress with a plaintive voice; and bewails himself in such melting music, that the whole neighbourhood sympathises with him in is sorrow' (Steele 1710, 158). In both examples—*Love by Love* and Steele's piece in *Tatler*—the word solo is reserved exclusively for the playing of music by an individual.

The definition of these words shows clear and careful differentiation. The *Oxford English Dictionary* defines the principal use of single as an adjective describing 'unaccompanied, individual; separate' (*OED*, s.v. "single"). Whereas, the principal definition for solo in the *Oxford English Dictionary* is for its use as a noun to mean '[s]enses relating to the performance by one person' as in music performed by an individual (*OED*, s.v. "solo").[5] By looking at the early applications of these words in written English, it is clear that the word single is loaded with negative connotations before even considering its connection with the historical shaming of women who conceive and birth outside marriage. Single has been used historically to highlight what a person lacks (such as worth in battle as in *Alexander and Dindimus*) and carries a stigma; solo, on the other hand, is more positively loaded because it highlights skill: in short, solo is an attribute but single is largely presented as a deficiency.[6]

With the mantle Single/Solo Mother by Choice, the addition of "choice" further complicates how single and solo mothers are linguistically framed. Arguably, one chooses to perform a solo but rarely would someone choose to be 'single by ourselves'. The association between solo and choice means that, almost by default, single becomes linked to unfortunate circumstance. In 'Mothering Alone: Rethinking Single Motherhood in America', Barbara Katz Rothman notes that it is largely unhelpful to differentiate based on this problematic notion of choice:

> [I]t is, I still think, about *raising children*. When you interview women who are doing that, it looks like it's about "motherhood." When you interview single women, it looks like it's about "single motherhood". (2009, 325)

Rothman argues that mothering has not changed dramatically but views on marriage have.[7] The SMBC is not a paradigm of the "anti"—anti-marriage, anti-men, anti-love, anti-romance—the SMBC is an icon of freedom afforded to women by advances in feminism as well as in the field of reproductive science. While this freedom is bound up in ideas of choice,

Rothman articulates the issue better when she speaks not of choice but of decisions: 'things happen; decisions get made that perhaps never were really "decisions," let alone "choices." Children happen. Mothers raise them' (2009, 328).

The idea of choice is nebulous from women choosing to parent solo after separating from a partner to women feeling they have no choice but to seek gamete donation and conceive before it is too late. I am sceptical of narratives that suggest, as Jean Renvoize describes in *Going Solo*, that 'the reality of single parenthood depends almost entirely on whether or not it was voluntary' (2023). What does it mean to volunteer for parenthood? Juffer notes that choice is actually the element that encompasses all mothers; she references television characters who are single mothers by choice—Rachel in *Friends* (1994–2004), who becomes pregnant by her ex-boyfriend and chooses to co-parent, as well as Miranda from *Sex and the City* (1998–2004), who decides against abortion when she becomes pregnant following a casual sexual relationship and chooses to become a single mother (2006, 1). These choices are arguably more authentic choices than, say, the choice of Emily from Robin Romm's *What to Expect*, whose agony over her donor pregnancy is rooted in her panic that she did not really want to choose solo motherhood at all.[8]

There is increasing attention to the problem of language with many mothers articulating a desire for less restrictive or stigmatised appellation. This is something Sarah Thompson in *Happy Single Mother* notes when she writes that she is a single mother but not always 'romantically unattached': 'it's hard to find the word for what I am. Single mother doesn't really cover it. I think I'd prefer independent mother, or something like that' (2023, 2–3). The cyborg might provide the answer. The cyborg represents the hybridisation of human and technology as well as a new language that challenges the binaries that have traditionally underpinned notions of identity. In this book, I have shown how these binaries are under pressure through the liminal experience of the SMBC who complicate the dualisms of man/woman, natural/artificial, mother/father in the traditional spaces of family, reproduction, and fertility through the use of assisted reproductive technologies to ironically conceive, birth and child rear solo. What this 'new language' should resist is becoming exclusionary. The SMBC as cyborg through mediated reproduction and through challenging traditional binaries should not exist in linguistic opposition to the single mother who is framed, by contrast, as somehow inferior.

The cyborg as a concept and entity is embedded within posthuman discourse. Although I read the posthuman—like many before me—as an ongoing development of the human condition, for many, the posthuman refers to a condition beyond human, with the prefix 'post' suggesting something that comes 'after'. N. Katherine Hayles explains why the 'post' in posthuman causes anxiety. Hayles remarks on the idea of human finality: '"Post," with its dual connotation of superseding the human and coming after it, hints that the days of "the human" might be numbered' (1999, 283). Although there are positives to posthumanism (to which Hayles subscribes), the fact remains that posthumanity is often understood as marking an 'end of a certain conception of the human' (1999, 286). The hybrid represents a possible melding of the traditional ways of understanding the human—such as human reproduction—and the proposition of a new way of negotiating human fundamentals such as conception and family construction. Many thinkers (such as Donna Haraway) would suggest this is evolutionary in terms of both our physical existence and in terms of social, political and cultural ways of understanding self in relation to technological structures and mediation. There is a risk that by dualistically separating single from solo mothering, solo mothers become framed as somehow 'post' single mother and therefore as a "betterment" or "advancement". I agree with scholars like Bock (2000) who argue that SMBC should include other single mother groups. But to be more precise, I believe the term solo mother should be encompassing. This is not to suggest a flattening out of experiences, but instead to prevent the gatekeeping of the term solo which is less burdened linguistically and historically. The solo mother should be a hybrid rather than a purity of concept.

The unification of single and solo mothers under the one term solo mother does not eradicate the complex social, cultural and economic issues impacting different family arrangements (including women with co-parents, women with known donors, women with anonymous donors, women solo parenting but romantically attached, women parenting in blended families, widows, divorcees, and so forth), but what it does do is combat a history and language which present single mothers as weak, vulnerable and worthless. Furthermore, avoiding the suffix "by choice" prevents implying that other one-parent families are victim to circumstance. Transparency of family origins is crucial to the development of healthy and well-adjusted offspring and so openness about gamete donation is important. It is for these reasons that I argue, as did the working group for *Independent Family Planning*, that Solo Parent (with the optional) via Donation (SPD) suffix offers better transparency and clarity (donation is a clearer pathway than choice) while resisting the diametrical othering of other women and different family types.

REFLECTION

Throughout the years, the words single and solo have evolved and now, in our contemporary, they are used interchangeably to mean 'alone'. But, going solo and being single do not mean being alone. As Ana Bravo-Moreno argues: 'the terms "single" and "solo" do not represent the experiences of the majority of women interviewed for whom family, friends, social networks, and community groups are important' (2019, 10). I was fortunate enough to find myself not only ushered into a community in which my children will be raised alongside other donor-conceived children and alongside other solo-parent families, but to find that fellow parents rallied around—solo mothers (by donation, through separation, through divorce, or widowed) and couples as well.

When, at thirty-one weeks, I went into premature labour I spoke on the phone to Anne-Marie for the very first time. I "met" Anne-Marie years before on a TV forum where we discussed, exclusively, science fiction shows. I had her phone number because when the forum became disused, we communicated through WhatsApp. I did not know a lot about her other than that she was a paediatrician in America. When I was unexpectedly sent down to the Labour and Delivery ward in Basildon Hospital, I panicked and called her. I had gone in for a routine appointment but was told the terrifying news that I was going to deliver my twins that day—two months early. I was bombarded with information and was in total shock. In desperation, I called the only medical doctor I knew—my sci-fi-loving buddy from America. That day was the first time I had ever heard her soothing west coast accent. When I dialled, I prayed she would answer the phone, and she did.

It was when I was in the NICU that I came to really know Stephanie. Stephanie and her husband—people I had met only twice before—sent me a bag full of clothes for premature babies—washed and ironed. Stephanie had experienced the NICU with her own twins and she was by the phone every day and helped me survive the NICU experience. Gently, she explained—before the nurses could—what I would see in the NICU, what the machines would be doing, and what to expect on the intensive care journey. Mostly, she sent me hope, company, and love. Then there was

Kayleigh, a solo mum who sat next to me in the NICU with her own baby. We supported each other as heart monitors beeped and the CPAP machines filled our friendly silences with white noise. Once home, miles away from each other, Kayleigh and I kept in contact through phone calls and text messages. Flicking back through messages over the last four years, I'm struck by the number of times we congratulated each other on little triumphs. The following exchange makes me smile—this is the text I sent Kayleigh the first time I took my babies out in the pram:

> 16 April 2019
> Me: I went outside!
> Kayleigh: Ahh yay well done x

Lauren, someone I had considered to be an acquaintance, popped over to see my newborns and then helped me breastfeed because it wasn't going quite right. Lauren—once a Facebook friend—is now a huge part of my life. Some friends from "before" drifted away, but new ones rose from the most unlikely places. I'm fortunate to know other solo mothers with whom I talk daily—the women interviewed here: Alexis, Eleni, Michelle, Nicola, Sam, Sarah A, Sarah B, Tamara, and Victoria and 50+ more on our local SMBC community group.

Through it all were my parents and brother James. My mum went to consultations and appointments with me—every single one. The four of us looked at donor profiles together and as a family team they helped me choose a donor we all thought sounded kind. My mum sat with me every day in the NICU, James ferried me back and forth, and dad made sure I had dinner when I got home. We merged homes during Covid so we could isolate without being isolated. My brother is now a live-in uncle, unbothered by toys all over the place and 6 am cacophony.

My children's godparents are vital people in our lives. Godmother Janine (Auntie Neen) is my oldest friend; she lives afar but always feels so close. Lee, the twins' Godfather and my best friend, proof-read this book (in fact he has read it several times over). Every Saturday at around 3 pm, my children squeal 'Uncle Lee!' in delight and run to the door. 'It's Uncle Lee, Uncle Lee is here!' He has been here throughout, and I know he will always be here.

I'm embedded in a long and fraught history of what it means to be a single woman; I'm a product of a feminist drive for reproductive freedom; I'm part of a complex debate on the nature of choice; I'm enveloped into a community of donor-conceived families; and I'm supported by a village of friends and family.

Maybe that's what it means to be cyborg: irretrievably enmeshed in technologies, people, and structures beyond oneself. Wholeness comprised of many parts. I'm a solo mother, I'm a donor recipient, I'm a one-parent family, and I'm a single woman outside of a relationship. I might be viewed as misguided, problematic, disadvantaged, feminist, determined, liberated, cyborgic.

What I'm not, however, is alone.

NOTES

1. Freezing eggs does not guarantee pregnancy. Freezing eggs later in life can mean freezing eggs with poor quality that might not be viable upon thawing and use.

2. Terminology is also important when it comes to speaking about and to donor-conceived offspring. The SMBC will use different language from the "single mother". Research suggests it is important for the word "donor" to be used with donor-conceived children rather than the words "father", "biological father", "birth father", "daddy", "dad". This is something Genevieve Roberts notes in her memoir: 'It's important to refer to the biological father as a donor, so that it does not set a child up with any false hopes that the donor will swoop in during adulthood as a daddy' (Roberts 2019, 48). Many SMBC books (e.g. Morrissette and Mattes) guide women through how to deal with the "where is my daddy?" question. This question is different for single mothers who will have to explain the absence (walkout, abandonment, new family, visitation, etc.), whereas the SMBC will answer 'our family does not have a daddy, instead we have a donor'. This does not mean the conversation is easier but it is categorically different. Naomi K. Cahn, writing on donor conception in America, states that 'The donor world is characterized by a vocabulary that serves as a cultural clue (cue) to our interpretation and understanding of these new families. The distinct linguistic choices show just what is at stake, and the syntax reflects broader questions about the donor world' (2013, 6). Here Cahn refers to how the words "donor", "sibling", and "mother" are used but—again—the differentiation between a single mother and solo mother is not considered despite the careful attention language is given by the donor conception society and industry.

3. Translation by Dr Isabel Davis.

4. There are different definitions and other contexts, but I am drawing on the earliest known uses. The intent here is to not provide an exhaustive overview of the evolution of these terms but to identify interesting elements about the origins.

5. As an adjective, sole is dated to 1386 and accredited to Geoffery Chaucer. The adjective was initially used to mean to 'live sole' and came to be principally defined as to mean unmarried. However, I did not include this term in the main body of the chapter as the use of "sole" to mean "unmarried" is now largely obsolete.

6. Single is not altogether a negative term; sport frequently refers to the single participant in tournaments and many creative hobbies are considered to be single pursuits, such as photography. Likewise, there are many exceptions in colloquial usage in which solo is used to mean to be alone—for example, to fly solo, to release a solo album, (etc.).

7. Mothering has changed in regard to what opportunities are now available to mothers and their offspring—for example, the introduction of free and funding-assisted childcare in the UK.

8. The way in which choice is privileged in some discourses on the single and solo mother is further problematised upon reflection that reproductive choice itself is increasingly under pressure. It has been made clear in some anti-donation bioethical discourse that some women are actively encouraged not to procreate. Now, the overturning of *Roe v. Wade* in America (June 24, 2022)—in which the US Supreme Court has granted individual states the right to limit or ban abortion—sees not only fifty years of Federal right to abortion abolished but actively calls into question the endurance of rights for non-traditional families and places under pressure bodily autonomy.

REFERENCES

Bock, J. D. 2000. Doing the Right Thing? Single Mothers by Choice and the Struggle for Legitimacy. *Gender and Society* 14(1): 62–86. http://www.jstor.org/stable/190422. Accessed March 4, 2021.

Bravo-Moreno, A. 2019. Deconstructing 'Single' Mothers by Choice: Transcending Blood, Genes, and the Biological Nuclear Family? *SAGE Open* 9(4). https://doi.org/10.1177/2158244019898258. Accessed November 15, 2023.

Cahn, N.R. 2009. *Test Tube Families. Why the Fertility Market Needs Legal Regulation*. New York: New York University Press.

———. 2013. *The New Kinship: Constructing Donor-Conceived Families*. London: New York University Press.

Congreve, W. (1695) 2010. *Love for Love*. ECCO.

Davis-Floyd, R., and J. Dumit, eds. 1998. *Cyborg Babies: From Techno-Sex to Techno-Tots*. London: Routledge.

Golombok, S., Zadeh, S., Freeman, T., Lysons, J., & Foley, S. 2021. Single Mothers by Choice: Parenting and Child Adjustment in Middle Childhood. *Journal of Family Psychology,* 35(2): 192–202. https://doi.org/10.1037/fam0000797. Accessed January 12, 2021.

Graham, S. 2012. Choosing Single Motherhood? Single Women Negotiating the Nuclear Family Ideal. In *Families—Beyond the Nuclear Ideal*, ed. Daniela Cutas and Sarah Chan, 97–109. London: Bloomsbury Academic.

———. 2018. Being a 'Good' Parent: Single Women Reflecting Upon 'Selfishness' and 'Risk' When Pursuing Motherhood Through Sperm Donation. *Anthropology & Medicine* 25: 249–264.

Halden, G., M. Johnson, S. Kamerkar, N. Milligan, G. Roberts, and R. Ward. 2023. *Independent Family Planning: Choosing Solo Motherhood through Gamete Donation. A Guide for Fertility Healthcare Professionals.* London: Wellcome.

Haraway, D. 1991. A Cyborg Manifesto: Science, Technology, and Socialist-Feminism in the Late Twentieth Century. In *Simians, Cyborgs, and Women: The Reinvention of the Nature*, 149–182. New York: Routledge.

Hayford, S.R., and K.B. Guzzo. 2015. The Single Mother by Choice Myth. *Contexts: Understanding People in Their Social Worlds* 14: 70–72.

Hayles, N.K. 1999. *How We Became Posthuman: Virtual Bodies in Cybernetics, Literature, and Informatics.* Chicago: University of Chicago Press.

Juffer, J. 2006. *Single Mother: The Emergence of the Domestic Individual.* London: New York University Press.

Mack, K. 2020. I Am Murphy Brown: Race and Class in Rhetorics of Single Mothers by Choice. *Rhetoric Review* 39 (3): 287–302.

Mattes, J. 1997. *Single Mothers by Choice: A Guidebook for Single Women Who Are Considering or Have Chosen Motherhood.* New York: Three Rivers Press.

Morrissette, M. 2008. *Choosing Single Motherhood: The Thinking Woman's Guide.* New York: Houghton Mifflin Company.

OED (*Oxford English Dictionary*. n.d. s.v. 'solo, n.1 and adj.' Accessed January 21 2021.

OED (*Oxford English Dictionary Online*). n.d. s.v. 'single, adj.' Accessed January 21, 2021.

Parke, R.D. 2013. *Future Families: Diverse Forms, Rich Possibilities.* Oxford: John Wiley & Sons.

Renvoize, J. 2023. *Going Solo: Single Mothers by Choice.* London: Routledge.

Roberts, G. 2019. *Going Solo: My Choice to Become a Single Mother Using a Donor.* London: Piatkus.

Rothman, B.K. 2009. Mothering Alone: Rethinking Single Motherhood in America. *WSQ: Women's Studies Quarterly* 37(2): 323–328. https://doi.org/10.1353/wsq.0.0199. Accessed March 17, 2023.

Steele, R. 1710. No 222. Saturday, September 9, 1710. In *The British Classics: Volume the Fourth. Containing the Fourth Volume of the Tatler* (C. Whittingham, 1804), pp. 154–158.

Thompson, S. 2023. *Happy Single Mother: Real Advice on How to Stay Sane and Why Things Aren't as Bad as You Think.* Thread.

Index[1]

---

[1] Note: Page numbers followed by 'n' refer to notes.

Printed by Printforce, United Kingdom